IMPROVE YOUR SMILE

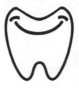

TRANSFORM YOUR LIFE

LESLIE PITNER, DDS, MS

IMPROVE YOUR SMILE

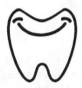

TRANSFORM YOUR LIFE

A GUIDE TO

ORTHODONTICS FOR ADULTS

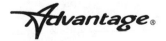

Published by Advantage, Charleston, South Carolina.
Member of Advantage Media Group.

ADVANTAGE is a registered trademark, and the Advantage colophon is a trademark of Advantage Media Group, Inc.

Printed in the United States of America.

ISBN: 978-1-59932-799-0
LCCN: 2016960883

Cover design by Katie Biondo.

This publication is designed to provide accurate and authoritative information in regard to the subject matter covered. It is sold with the understanding that the publisher is not engaged in rendering legal, accounting, or other professional services. If legal advice or other expert assistance is required, the services of a competent professional person should be sought.

Advantage Media Group is proud to be a part of the Tree Neutral® program. Tree Neutral offsets the number of trees consumed in the production and printing of this book by taking proactive steps such as planting trees in direct proportion to the number of trees used to print books. To learn more about Tree Neutral, please visit **www.treeneutral.com.**

Advantage Media Group is a publisher of business, self-improvement, and professional development books. We help entrepreneurs, business leaders, and professionals share their Stories, Passion, and Knowledge to help others Learn & Grow. Do you have a manuscript or book idea that you would like us to consider for publishing? Please visit **advantagefamily.com** or call **1.866.775.1696.**

TABLE OF CONTENTS

ABOUT THE AUTHOR

Dr. Leslie Pitner, DDS, MS, MAPP, attended Williams College, where she received her undergraduate degree in 1990. At Williams, she majored in art and graduated with highest honors, earning membership in Phi Beta Kappa. After completing a master's degree in art history at the University of Pennsylvania in 1995, she decided to pursue a career in dentistry. She graduated with distinction from the University of North Carolina (UNC) School of Dentistry in 2002, where she was elected to membership in Omicron Kappa Upsilon (OKU), a dental honor society. She also completed her specialty certificate at UNC and received her master of science in orthodontics in 2005. Beyond her technical training in dentistry and orthodontics, she also completed a unique master's degree program in positive psychology at the University of Pennsylvania in 2007. Positive psychology focuses on personal growth and happiness (rather than on pathology and mental illness) in human development.

Dr. Pitner has lectured on aesthetic orthodontics across the USA, with a focus on lingual braces. She has also lectured on the psychology of the smile, based on the original research she did for her master's degree in positive psychology. She continues to be active in teaching and research and, most recently, has given seminars at the UNC and the University of Illinois. She also serves on the board of reviewers for the *American Journal of Orthodontics and Dentofa-*

cial Orthopedics, the most prestigious scientific journal in the field of orthodontics.

Her practice, Pitner Orthodontics, offers three locations: two in Columbia, South Carolina, and one in Chapin, South Carolina. Her downtown Columbia office is the only orthodontic practice in the US purpose-built to exclusively serve adults.

ACKNOWLEDGMENTS

This book would not have been possible without the help of many people. The idea floated around in my head for almost ten years before it got to ink on paper. Thank you to Martin Seligman, the founder of the MAPP program at Penn, and my amazing diva friends (Karen, Gail, Joanna, Julie, and Ming) who encouraged me to pursue my interest in the psychology behind the smile and planted the first seed for this project. Thank you to Dr. William Proffit for teaching me that it takes a lot of knowledge to explain something simply. Thank you to my amazing team at Pitner Orthodontics for believing me and supporting me when I told them I was going to write a book. Thank you to Jenny Tripp and Scott Neville for helping me find my voice. And my final thank you is to the best writing teacher I ever had: my husband Kirk Kicklighter. This is dedicated to you and could never have happened without your unwavering belief that I can.

INTRODUCTION

Years ago I had sweet little Claire as a patient. She was a quiet girl who brought her teddy bear along to appointments. Much like Claire, her mother was the nicest person you'd ever meet, adorable and lively, like a ray of blonde sunshine. Mom called her daughter Claire Bear, and it fit her perfectly, save for one thing. Sweet as she was, the smile Claire had before we started her in braces did not fit her. Her teeth were crowded, her jaw was misaligned, and none of her front teeth touched. The day we took off Claire's braces, the change was remarkable. She had gone from having teeth splayed all over to having a lovely smile. Her mom looked at me in awe.

"You must have the best job in the world," she said. "You get to change people's lives."

She was right. I do! And the satisfaction I get from seeing my patients go from shy and self-effacing to radiantly self-confident never gets old. When you've spent most of your life hiding your smile or just stopped smiling altogether because you're embarrassed by your teeth, it's amazing what happens when your braces come off. Suddenly, you feel great about yourself, confident in meeting others, free to laugh and talk and enjoy yourself without that nagging fear that people will be put off by what they see when they look at you. It's literally a life-changing experience, and it doesn't matter how old you are. I've had patients in their seventies and older who've said,

"This is the best thing I've ever done for myself." Their only regret is not having done it sooner.

As much as I love what I do, I didn't always see my career path so clearly. Frankly, I was a reluctant orthodontist. When I applied for my orthodontic residency, that time in their career when orthodontic students insist they always wanted to be an orthodontist, my first line was "I *never* wanted to be an orthodontist." The funny thing was that everything I'd done before then made it a perfect fit for me, but I didn't see it coming.

My dad was an orthodontist back in the day when orthodontists didn't wear gloves. So, as a kid, I thought his putting his hands in someone else's mouth had to be the singularly most disgusting thing anyone could possibly do. There was absolutely no way I was going to do that. Added to that, everyone in my father's family worked in the sciences. I wasn't going to make science a career. Nope. Not me. I was going to be creative. I just didn't know quite how.

I stumbled into art history when I was a sophomore at Williams College. I hadn't been aware that such a thing as an art history major existed—until I took an introductory class on architecture and sculpture. Suddenly I was thinking and writing about things that were real and three-dimensional, and the light bulb went on. I'd considered becoming an English major, but writing about beautiful things, and the relationships between objects and the space around them, seemed so much more meaningful. Then putting them into the context of the times in which they were created—wow! This was heady stuff to me! I majored in art history, loved it, and decided to pursue a PhD after college.

I completed my master's degree and started looking ahead to an academic career. The problem was that the closer I came to becoming an academic, the less sure I was that it was the right profession for me. I'd stuck it out in grad school for as long as I had thanks to a multiyear fellowship that made it tough to quit. But there was a problem: I couldn't stand to read one more thing about art, art history, or architecture. What had once fascinated me now seemed too abstract and impractical.

I was in grad school at the University of Pennsylvania, and my new husband was up at Harvard, so I moved to Boston to be with him and, ostensibly, to prepare for my PhD exams. The plan was that I'd study at the architecture library there, where I'd have all the resources of the world at my fingertips. Instead, I spent my days thumbing through the magazine collections and drinking coffee.

When I went to take my PhD oral exam, I flopped spectacularly. I can laugh about it now, but at the time, it was humiliating. I knew I had it coming, though. Given my total lack of preparation, it was the logical outcome. In fact, there was a moment during the exam when I nearly said, "You know what? It's clear that I have no idea what I'm talking about, and I am not prepared at all, so why don't we just stop?" I wish I had. My advisor found me afterward and told me I had failed. I hadn't needed to be told, but it made it official. My peers were horrified, and I enjoyed the momentary notoriety of being the first person in anyone's memory to have failed the oral exam. I probably should have been ashamed, but I felt I had been released from prison. Now it was finally time to reassess and think about what I really wanted to do with my life.

It occurred to me that I should go to medical school. But I still loved the visual part of art study, how beautiful things are constructed, how they make a difference in our lives, and how we interact with them. So I told my father in all seriousness, "Maybe being a radiologist would be like being an art historian—because I would still be interpreting pictures—but more useful." At that moment, that made perfectly good sense.

My dad looked thoughtful. "Why don't you think about dental school?" My initial response was a shrug, but he kept going. "Talk to some dentists. Talk to some physicians. Just see how it feels." That was great advice because I started talking to doctors and volunteering at hospitals and realized I didn't like being around sick people. (I know this makes me a bad person, but there you go.) At the same time, I talked to people working in dentistry, and everyone I talked to seemed to love it. The more I learned about it, the more attractive I found the work. It was meaningful—I would be helping people—it was aesthetic, and it was real and concrete. I'd be replacing something, fixing something, and making something more beautiful—all the things I enjoyed doing in one practical package. And orthodontics was the most appealing specialty because thinking and planning was involved, creating and executing a strategy that takes time and skill to achieve the desired results. I remember telling a fellow student at dental school why that attracted me. He shook his head and said, "I can't imagine doing that. That's like taking care of a bonsai tree. You have to be very patient." That was true, and that was part of what I liked about it. He wound up as an orthodontist too, with his own little "bonsai farm."

Still, it wasn't until I got through dental school and was in my residency at the University of North Carolina, actually doing orthodontics, that I realized what a perfect fit this career was for me. Back when I was at Penn, I had audited a class on abnormal psychology led by Professor Martin Seligman, the author of a bestselling book titled *Learned Optimism*. His class planted in me a seed of interest in psychology that I followed up in my orthodontics residency by writing a thesis tied to the topic. I was interested in the notion of self-efficacy, the idea that what you *will* do is based on your beliefs about what you *can* do. When I was doing research for my thesis, I discovered that Professor Seligman was starting a new program at Penn, a master's degree in applied positive psychology. Initially, the idea of taking on yet more schooling was not attractive, but I had the flexibility to do it, and about a year after hearing about the program, I decided to go ahead and earn that degree. It was there that I dove deep into the research that would lead to my thesis on the psychology behind the smile. You'll learn more about that in the first chapter and how important smiling is, not just for how others perceive us but also for our self-esteem, our mental and physical health, and even our longevity.

Mine was a circuitous path, but when you think about it, it all fits. Taken together, the areas I've explored give me a genuinely holistic grasp of orthodontics, and that's valuable to my patients because I can tell them *why*. If you want to know why it's important that your teeth fit together from a functional perspective, I can describe that for you. If you want me to tell you how smiling is going to affect your brain, how you see yourself, and how you respond to other people, I can clarify that. If you want to know exactly how your smile is going to affect how other people see you, their perceptions of you, and how intelligent or successful you are, I can explain the science of that as well. All of those factors are tied to your smile, and they're all hugely important.

But to me, the most important piece is the one that came out of my studies in positive psychology: the concept of an upward spiral of positive emotions. The psychologist Barbara Fredrickson studied how the experience of positive emotions changes our brain and how we interact with others in a process she called broaden and build. Positive emotions generate receptivity, an openness to learning, to new people, and to new experiences. That brings you more knowledge and more skills and builds upon itself to create an upward spiral toward ever-greater positivism. A beautiful smile—where one had once been missing—can be the key to creating a new upward spiral. A smile with crooked teeth, one that undermines your confidence, creates a downward spiral that you probably are not even aware of.

How does this downward spiral happen? If you feel uncomfortable smiling when you meet new people, for example, others are likely to see you as less friendly and approachable. Have you trained yourself to cock your head in a particular way when your picture is taken to avoid emphasizing a protruding tooth? Do you turn down opportunities at work because you wonder if people will judge your smile? Do you make sure to cover your mouth when you laugh? How many actions do you reflexively perform every day to compensate for an imperfection in your smile?

I've helped my patients learn how to smile again, literally, after a lifetime of covering their unattractive teeth. I've seen the impact the upward spiral of a new confident smile has had on their relationships, their careers, and their self-esteem.

That's why I wrote this book.

Your smile and how you feel about it isn't a small thing. It's a *gigantic* thing—and it's not just for kids. Perhaps getting your teeth fixed is something you've always meant to do but never quite got around to. Maybe you got in the habit of putting everyone's needs or wants ahead of yours, and now you feel as though it's too late to make a difference. Or maybe you were fortunate enough to have braces early in life, and so you avoided the shame and embarrassment of having ugly teeth as a teenager, but your teeth have slowly shifted over the years.

Whether it's been a lifetime or just a few years, you need to know that it doesn't have to be that way. You can give yourself a life-changing, lifelong gift—and I promise it will be quicker, more comfortable, and less awkward than you think it's going to be.

At this point, part of you may be dismissing the idea of an improved smile as mere cosmetics or simple vanity. But it's so much bigger and more profound than that. In the chapters to come, I'll share the research that evidences the power of a smile, and I'll discuss how a smile changes us inside and out. I'll explore the myths you may hold about orthodontics and explain the processes, options, and advances in technology that have made so much more possible today than in the past. I think you will find that orthodontic treatment is much easier and more convenient than you imagine.

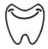

CHAPTER ONE

THE SCIENCE BEHIND YOUR SMILE

"Doctor Pitner, I'm about a year away from retirement, and I don't want to go on to the next phase of my life looking like this. I want to be able to smile without worrying what people will think of me. Can you help me, or did I wait too long?"

My first impression of Pam was that of an attractive, well-dressed lady in her late middle years. She rose gracefully to meet me as I came into the waiting room. But she wasn't smiling, and that's always a bad sign. When she spoke, I could see why her smile was missing in action. Her teeth were like a laundry list of things gone wrong. With a deep overbite, teeth badly discolored with gaps where some were missing or crooked, and old, ill-fitting bridgework, her mouth certainly did not match the pride she took in the rest of her appearance. Clearly, this lady needed to get her smile back, and I knew I could help her.

How important is a smile to how we feel and how others see us?

In a word, crucial. There are many different expressions that communicate negative emotions—sadness, fear, anger, disgust—but the smile is the single human expression that tells others we're happy, friendly, or content. For this reason alone, the smile plays an unparalleled role in our emotions and communication with others. The true, genuine smile is unmistakable. It creates an authentic connection between people. On the other hand, we can instinctively spot a fake, forced, or pained smile.

Dr. Guillaume-Benjamin-Amand Duchenne (de Boulogne) was a nineteenth-century French neurologist whose groundbreaking research on facial expressions revealed the complex relationship between facial muscles working together to produce a genuine smile, as opposed to the grimace you make when you just lift the corners of your mouth. An authentic smile is a reflex completely tied into the experience of happiness and joy. Our brain creates this smile, but even more amazing is the fact that the act of smiling actually creates a neurological feedback loop that, in turn, *makes you feel happier*.

Dr. Duchenne made a significant contribution to our understanding of facial expressions. He was the first to systematically investigate which muscles were involved in making each individual expression. Almost by accident, he discovered that, physiologically, there are two distinct types of smiles. He found that what we recognize as an authentic smile arises from the activation of not only the zygomatic (cheek raising) muscle but also the orbicularis oculi muscles of the eyes, so that smiling faces not only show teeth but also have a distinctive crinkling around the eyes. (They're not called laugh lines for nothing!)[1]

When people only activate the zygomatic muscles, revealing their teeth, they have a "grin-and-bear-it" facial expression, which is not at all like the spontaneous smile elicited by a joke or a pleasurable experience. Even though Duchenne's work was lost for over a century, he has been memorialized for his discovery of the authentic smile. The authentic smile, which activates both the zygomatic and orbicularis oculi muscles, is now dubbed the Duchenne smile.

ARE SMILES UNIVERSAL?

We now know that the recognition of genuine (versus social or forced) smiles is universal across cultures, but it took over one hundred years of scientific debate to reach that conclusion. In the nineteenth century, after Duchenne, Charles Darwin was the first scientist inspired to tackle the meaning of facial expressions, dedicating a book to the subject.[2] His idea was that expressions have a biological basis and are the same for all humans. But by the 1950s, Darwin's ideas had fallen out of favor as major anthropologists, such as Margaret Mead, argued that facial expressions were not universal but were culturally conditioned. These scholars believed that people learned through social experience that a smile meant happy and a grimace meant sad and that no expression was hardwired.

Then, in 1965, a young psychologist named Paul Ekman, who was studying nonverbal behavior, decided to challenge Mead. To do it right, he needed to study a group of people who had virtually no contact with any other culture in the world. He traveled to Papua New Guinea to live with the Fore tribe, whose nearly complete isolation from the outside world made them ideal subjects for study. He found a few boys who had been taught English by missionaries to serve as his translators. His first experiment was to show the tribesmen a series of photographs of people making discrete facial expressions (e.g., smiling or showing surprise, fear, anger, etc.), and he asked them to tell a story based on each facial expression. What he quickly found was that the Fore tribesmen recognized what the facial expressions meant, even on Western faces they were not accustomed to. He then had the tribesmen read a story and choose the photo of a facial expression that expressed the story. Again, they all chose the correct expression. Finally, he told simple stories—such as a story about someone who's happy because his friends have come to visit—to members of the tribe and asked them to make a facial expression that fit the story. Again, they made the same facial expressions that we'd all recognize and understand. Ekman realized that the previously accepted conclusions of scholars—that facial expressions are culturally determined and not hardwired—was completely wrong.[3] He had discovered his life's work as an expert on facial expressions.

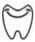

"Sometimes, your joy is the source of your smile, but sometimes, your smile can be the source of your joy."
—Thich Nhat Hanh

CAN SMILING MAKE YOU HAPPIER?

What comes first, smiling or feeling happy? Can the act of smiling itself—in the absence of a reason to smile—make a person feel good?

Paul Ekman joined with Richard Davidson, one of the world's experts on the neuroscience of emotions, to study this question. They found students who were able to produce a true enjoyment smile on command and hold that smile for at least twenty seconds. The brain activity of these students was measured while they exhibited true enjoyment smiles versus mere social smiles. Ekman and Davidson found that the act of voluntarily producing a Duchenne smile—even with no emotional trigger—activated the left frontal portion of the brain, the very same part of the brain activated during the experience of real happiness, contentment, and joy.[4] In other words, smiling may not make you happy when you are having a really bad day, but it can help make a so-so day good or a good day great. The idea of fake it 'til you make it is not so far-fetched.

SHINY HAPPY PEOPLE—SO WHAT?

So why should we care? What does feeling contentment or happiness do for people? Do positive emotions have any real purpose at all? While humans have long been occupied with the definition of happiness and have devoted endless books, philosophies, and religions to achieving happiness, we have not always been very clear about *why* we should feel happy. Until the past decade, happiness and positive emotions were the orphaned children of psychology. Psychologists had developed well-established theories to explain the purpose of negative emotions such as fear (to get us to run the other way fast) or anger (to get ready to fight). But more recently, scientists are discovering that a feeling of happiness does so much more than create a good feeling. The evidence from studies of individuals and groups is becoming overwhelming that positive emotions, facial expressions, moods, and traits lead to many positive outcomes. Good feelings cause people to be more creative and open-minded and improve their health, and they may even delay death. A recent analysis of over 250 studies investigating positive affect (e.g., smiling, good mood, feelings of happiness) found evidence that happiness leads to success, not the other way around.[5] Such results argue that happy people have or develop resources that help them find their way to good jobs, good marriages, good friends, and good health.

SMILING AS A PREDICTOR OF FUTURE HAPPINESS

What if a single photograph of a true enjoyment smile could predict how happy and confident a person will feel over twenty-five years later? One particularly intriguing study did just that. Researchers looked at college yearbook photos of students from a small women's college and evaluated the women's facial expressions to see whether they displayed a Duchenne (enjoyment) smile.[6] These same women were followed for over twenty-five years, completing various psychological questionnaires and describing their life circumstances at the age of twenty-seven, forty-three, and fifty-two. The young women who had smiled in the yearbook photos were initially described as having more warmth and personal charm. Over time, they also became more competent, experienced fewer negative emotions, were more likely to be happily married, and were more satisfied with their lives. It seems remarkable that a single photograph of a true smile could give a snapshot of the future, but, in fact, that single image does demonstrate the power of a genuine smile of happiness.

YOUR SMILE ON THE JOB

It makes sense that smiling and feeling good would affect close personal relationships, but does it make any difference in the dog-eat-dog world of work? The answer is yes. Smiling can change not only how satisfied individuals are with their work but also how well they perform and are evaluated by managers and coworkers. Workers who are happier and more satisfied with their lives get better job performance feedback than those with low positive affect.[7] Managers who were rated by observers as having more positive affect achieved better performances on an objective test of their managerial skills.[8] Smiling and feeling positive emotions also has long-term effects on job success. Employees of three different companies were interviewed by trained surveyors and completed a questionnaire about depression, happiness at work, and physical energy.[9] The employees were also observed at work and scored on how often they smiled, laughed, or said something funny. Eighteen months later, the researchers gathered information on job evaluations, pay, and social support at work. The people who were happier in their work and smiled more often were rated more highly by their supervisors, earned higher pay, and enjoyed more social support from their supervisor and coworkers.

Having positive emotions improves performance not only for individuals but also for groups. Work teams with a positive outlook have been shown to be more successful on the job. High-performing and low-performing work groups were observed for their team dynamics by researchers who noted the amount of positive versus negative interaction. The researchers found that the highest-performing teams had a ratio of about 5:1 positive to negative interactions while lowest-performing teams had a ratio of less than 1:1.[10] The expression of positive emotions such as encouragement and support made for more successful work teams and not just on an interpersonal level. These teams were more profitable, had better customer ratings, and were more admired by colleagues.

SMILING GETS YOU HIRED

In fact, some interviewers use rating systems to winnow out the nonsmilers. One national hotel chain's human resources department literally counted the number of times that interviewees smiled during their interviews. Candidates who smiled fewer than four times didn't make it to the next round. The Greyhound Bus Company used the same kind of metric. A candidate had to smile at least five times during a fifteen-minute interview to get a job. Smiling gets you higher tips too. According to an experiment conducted in a Seattle cocktail bar in 1978, a waitress's genuine smile brought her double the tips she earned when she didn't smile.[11]

SMILING MAY EVEN MAKE US SMARTER

Why do positive emotions and smiles create more success at work? There is strong evidence that feeling good makes people smarter and more creative. Alice Isen has been at the vanguard of research in this area. She has shown that positive feelings, whether inspired by a gift of candy or watching a funny movie, lead people to be more flexible in how they think and help them to arrive at correct answers to complex problems more quickly.[12] In one of her best-known studies, experienced physicians were given a small bag of candy, given nothing, or asked to read a series of statements about the medical profession.[13] The physicians were then asked to determine the diagnosis of a complex medical case. The doctors who were given the candy arrived at the correct diagnosis almost twice as fast as the other two groups.

A similar result has been found in young children who were given a task from the Wechsler Intelligence Scale for Children (WISC), the test used to determine the IQ of children.[14] After listening to stories that ended on either a happy or sad note, the children worked on puzzles from the WISC. The children who had listened to the happy story completed 50 percent more of the problems correctly and finished more quickly. This result seems even more remarkable when you consider that these children were that much more successful on the very test that establishes IQ! Clearly, feeling happy really can make you smarter.

SMILING PEOPLE LIVE LONGER

Can feeling positive emotions actually help you to live longer? One remarkable study suggests just that. Retired nuns aged 75 to 102 were part of a landmark study on aging and Alzheimer's disease. Many of these women had written short autobiographies when they first took their vows. Researchers coded these autobiographies for positive and negative emotional content.[15] Expressions of emotion such as happiness, love, or gratitude were coded as positive, while others such as sadness, fear, and suffering were coded as negative. They discovered:

1. The happiest nuns lived ten years longer than the least happy nuns.

2. By the age of eighty, the happiest group had only lost 25 percent of its population while the least happy group had lost 60 percent.

3. The happiest nuns had an 80 percent chance of getting to the age of eighty-five while the least cheerful nuns only had a 54 percent chance of reaching eighty-five years of age.

4. The happiest ninety-year-old nuns had a 65 percent probability of living longer, while the least happy ninety-year-old sisters had only a 30 percent probability of living longer.

5. Fifty-four percent of the happiest nuns reached the age of ninety-four, while only 15 percent of the least happy nuns reached that age.

These results are even more remarkable when you consider how homogenous this group of women was. They had all been teachers until their retirement, were well educated, lived in similar environments, and, of course, were unmarried.

In another study titled *Smile Intensity in Photographs Predicts Longevity*, Wayne State University researchers used baseball cards to analyze the smiles of 230 Major League Baseball players from the 1952 player register.[16] The study included controls for body mass index, the length of their careers, their marital status, and their education. The researchers sorted the photos into categories: no smile, partial smile, and the Duchenne smile. And guess what? On average, the nonsmilers lived to be 72.9 years old, while the partial smilers lived to 75 years, and the Duchenne smilers lived to 79.9 years.

SMILING FACES ARE SEEN AS MORE ATTRACTIVE

In a research paper titled *Beauty in a Smile*, researchers revealed the results of a study of brain response in people viewing attractive faces. The attractive faces displayed either neutral expressions or smiles.[17] The study found that attractive faces, in general, activated in observers the part of the brain associated with rewards, but smiling, attractive faces got a much greater response in the observer's brain. Our brains see a smiling face as a bigger reward.

Now you understand why a smile's a terrible thing to hide (or lose)!

The evidence is overwhelming. A smile has a huge impact on the smiler's life in ways both obvious and completely unexpected. It goes far beyond mere aesthetics or vanity. And clearly, a lot depends on how others judge us from our smiles. You don't have to be a scientist to figure that out.

I once treated a bright, personable, young salesman in his twenties, who had decided to get braces because he knew his discomfort—due to his smile—in making business presentations was damaging his career and preventing him from moving up the ladder. His teeth were quite crowded, with some hidden behind others, making him look as if he were missing a front tooth. I knew I could help, and in two years he went from being the guy who always avoided the limelight to someone with a winning smile worthy of his endearing personality. His confidence soared so much that he now *volunteers* to give presentations, and his bosses have taken notice.

Here's another example. Perhaps the biggest personality change I have ever seen occurred in a quiet, sweet-natured man whose underbite made him look like a cranky bulldog. Rob was a subdued guy whose wife did most of his talking for him in our initial meeting. Several orthodontists had already told him nothing could be done for him, and I got the sense that Rob had only agreed to see me at his wife's insistence. Clearly, she wanted a transformation for him, and I was happy to tell them both that, yes, I could help. His case was challenging, but he was a great sport about it, and within three or four months, I saw a huge change in the appearance of his teeth. But what astonished me was how much his personality shifted. He went from being nearly mute to being the guy who came in smiling and chatting with everyone in the reception area. He even got his hair tipped blonde like Guy Fieri! The alteration in his self-confidence was night and day. He was so happy with the changes he'd seen and how he felt about himself that his joy made our staff beam with gratitude for the work we are privileged to do for others. He became one of our most favorite patients ever.

Truth be told, so many of our patients begin treatment as Pam did—Pam is the lady I told you about at the beginning of this chapter. These patients have literally forgotten how to smile after years of reflexively contorting their facial expressions to conceal their unattractive teeth. *But they learn fast!* Pam stopped by to visit me not long ago, and when I asked her how she liked her new looks, she beamed. "Dr. Pitner," she said, "I have the prettiest smile in town and I love to share it!"

Your smile is *that* important. It makes *that* kind of difference in your life.

CHAPTER ONE NOTES

1   G.-B. Duchenne de Boulogne, *The Mechanism of Human Facial Expression, Studies in Emotion and Social Interaction*, ed. P. Ekman and K. R. Scherer (1862, repr. Cambridge: Cambridge University Press, 1990).

2   C. Darwin, *The Expression of Emotions in Man and Animals* (1872, repr. Oxford: Oxford University Press, 2002).

3   P. Ekman, *Emotions Revealed* (New York: Owl Books, 2003).

4   R. J. Davidson et al., "Approach-Withdrawal and Cerebral Asymmetry: Emotional Expression and Brain Physiology: I," *Journal of Personality and Social Psychology* 58, no. 2 (1990): 330–341.

5   S. Lyubomirsky, L. King, and E. Diener, "The Benefits of Frequent Positive Affect: Does Happiness Lead to Success?" *Psychological Bulletin* 131, no. 6 (2005): 803–855.

6   L. Harker and D. Keltner, "Expressions of Positive Emotion in Women's College Yearbook Pictures and Their Relationship to Personality and Life Outcomes across Adulthood," *Journal of Personality & Social Psychology* 80, no.1 (2001): 112–124.

7   R. Cropanzano and T. A. Wright, "A 5-Year Study of Change in the Relationship between Well-Being and Job Performance," *Consulting Psychology Journal: Practice and Research* 51 (1999): 252–265.

8   B. M. Staw and S. G. Barsade, "Affect and Managerial Performance: A Test of the Sadder-but-Wiser vs. Happier-and-Smarter Hypothesis," *Administrative Science Quarterly* 38 (1993): 304–331.

9   B. M. Staw, R. I. Sutton, and L. H. Pelled, "Employee Positive Emotion and Favorable Outcomes at the Workplace," *Organization Science* 5 (1994): 51–71.

10   B. L. Fredrickson and M. F. Losada, "Positive Affect and the Complex Dynamics of Human Flourishing," *American Psychologist* 60, no. 7 (2005): 678–686.

11   M. LaFrance, *Lip Service: Smiles in Life, Death, Trust, Lies, Work, Memory, Sex, and Politics* (New York: W. W. Norton, 2011).

12   A. M. Isen, "An Influence of Positive Affect on Decision Making in Complex Situations: Theoretical Issues with Practical Implications," *Journal of Consumer Psychology* 11, no. 2 (2001): 75–85.

13   C. A. Estrada, A. M. Isen, and M. J. Young, "Positive Affect Facilitates Integration of Information and Decreases Anchoring in Reasoning among Physicians," *Organizational Behavior and Human Decision Processes* 72, no. 1 (1997): 117–135.

14   N. Rader and E. Hughes, "The Influence of Affective State on the Performance of a Block Design Task in 6- and 7-Year-Old Children," *Cognition & Emotion* 19 no. 1 (2005): 143–150.

15   D. D. Danner, D. A. Snowdon, and W. V. Friesen, "Positive Emotions in Early Life and Longevity: Findings from the Nun Study," *Journal of Personality and Social Psychology* 80, no. 5 (2001): 804–813.

16   E. L. Abel and M. L. Kruger, "Smile Intensity in Photographs Predicts Longevity," *Psychological Science* 21, no. 4 (2010): 542–544.

17   J. O'Doherty et al., "Beauty in a Smile: The Role of Medial Orbitofrontal Cortex in Facial Attractiveness," *Neuropsychologia,* special issue, *The Cognitive Neuroscience of Social Behavior* 41, no. 2 (2003): 147–155.

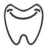

CHAPTER TWO

ORTHODONTIC MYTHS BUSTED

"Why does she need braces? Why can't we just pull that tooth that isn't coming in right?"

It wasn't the first time he'd asked me this, and I wondered yet again what in the world this obviously caring father was thinking. His daughter had an impacted canine, a tooth that was not coming into place properly on its own. She would need braces to pull it into place, but for an orthodontist, this was completely routine. "She's going to need that tooth," I explained for the umpteenth time. "That canine has an important job to do and I can easily bring it into place."

What keeps people from seeking orthodontic treatment? Sometimes, it's fear: they remember the bad old days when braces made your mouth look like the grille on a '57 Chevy and were about as comfortable. Things have changed for the better since then, but some folks haven't heard the news.

In this case, I'd been checking this young lady's teeth every year for four or five years and could see that they were crowded and this one wasn't coming in properly. Every year, her father and I sat down to discuss her case, and every time I mentioned bringing the canine in, he dug in his heels: "Why can't we just take that tooth out?"

That's when I finally asked him, "Tell me what it is you're so worried about."

He said, "Aren't you going to have to tie her top teeth to her bottom teeth to be able to do that? When I was a kid I had to have the same thing done and they tied that top tooth to my bottom teeth." To this day I still have no idea what kind of procedure he was talking about, but he had the idea that we were basically going to wire his daughter's mouth shut. No wonder he was worried!

That wasn't my first experience, or my last, with the odd ideas some people have about how we move teeth. I doubt what the father remembered was what had really happened to him, but it was clearly his perception, and he wasn't about to inflict such an experience on his daughter. Once I was able to reassure him that her treatment was going to be straightforward and easy, he was totally on board. I always recall that case when I encounter people whose mistaken assumptions or expectations make them resist doing something that's actually pretty easy because they think it's going to be a whole lot harder and more painful than it really is.

In this chapter, I want to counter some of the common misconceptions I run into and provide you with a better understanding of how orthodontics work, in hopes of reassuring those of you who are hesitant to seek treatment.

"BRACES ARE JUST FOR KIDS."

One quarter of the people getting orthodontic treatment in the United States are adults, and that number continues to climb as treatment becomes easier and the options more aesthetic. Many people assume that adult teeth are harder (or impossible) to move, and I think that many orthodontists have contributed to that notion by their disinclination to take on adult patients. In fact, any adult's teeth can be moved just as easily as a child's can. I have treated patients in their eighties, and many of my patients are in their forties, fifties, and sixties. Their kids have grown up and moved out, so the parents finally have the time and money to take care of themselves, and they've decided to get their teeth fixed.

Another thing to consider is that we're living longer and people are keeping their teeth for a lifetime. People used to think, *Yes, my teeth are ugly, but I'm going to end up with dentures anyway.* Very few of us will end up with dentures these days. Some of us assume we'll just stop caring about our appearance at some point down the line, but in my experience, if you don't like your smile, it's not going to stop bothering you just because you're getting older. In fact, the older you get, the better you're going to want to feel about yourself—and your smile is a great place to start.

"I HAVE TO BE REFERRED TO AN ORTHODONTIST."

The myth here is that if your dentist doesn't refer you, you can't or don't need to see an orthodontist, and that's completely untrue. Many dentists don't recommend orthodontics unless there is a serious bite problem or some other noncosmetic issue. And even then, they may not refer a patient, because they assume that adults don't want or need braces. Add to this that we've been conditioned by the medical system to assume we need a referral when it comes to seeing a specialist, but that isn't so when it comes to orthodontics. There's no gatekeeper; you can make the decision on your own, and it won't affect your insurance if you have coverage.

"I'LL BE IN THE OFFICE WITH A BUNCH OF TWELVE-YEAR-OLDS."

This may be true in many orthodontic practices, but increasingly, orthodontists are seeing the need to create a different experience for their adult patients. Look for orthodontists who treat a number of adults, who seem comfortable when they meet you, and who have a location that's dedicated to adults or at least a portion of their office set aside for adults, whether that's a separate reception area or a separate treatment area. Not everyone minds being around kids, of course, but many practices are set up to cater mostly to kids' specific needs and hours, and those hours don't necessarily accommodate working adults. Find a practice that does because the more orthodontists have worked with adults, the better they will be at addressing your unique concerns. Kids tend to be more compliant and less questioning than adults, and frankly, some practitioners prefer that. You need to find someone who's going to be willing to take the extra time to listen to your thoughts, address your questions, and keep you informed about where you are in your treatment.

"BRACES TAKE TOO LONG. I'LL BE WEARING THEM FOR YEARS."

Most patients vastly overestimate the time it will take to fix their teeth. Depending on how complicated things are, on average, most treatment takes somewhere from about six months to two years. I've had people tell me that they were in braces for five years when they were kids. I don't know whether that's true, but it certainly must have seemed that long to them! Treatment did take longer in the past than it does today, but now it can be accelerated thanks to new technologies and materials.

"I DON'T HAVE TIME FOR ORTHODONTICS. I'D HAVE TO BE IN YOUR OFFICE EVERY OTHER WEEK OR ONCE A MONTH FOR CHECKUPS."

This is totally untrue. In fact, I see most of my patients at six-week to ten-week intervals. Most of the subsequent appointments after the initial one are relatively brief, anywhere from ten to thirty minutes long. Sometimes, people tell me they'd come in more often if that would speed up their treatment, and I have to tell them that's not how it works. (See chapter four to learn about the biology that makes this true.)

"ARE YOU GOING TO CRANK MY BRACES?"

This sounds like something out of the Spanish Inquisition, but many people have asked me this question. Some of them may have had (or had a friend who had) an expander, an oral appliance that is turned with a key and feels as if it is being cranked. But this idea probably also comes from forty to fifty years ago when the stiff, stainless-steel wires would initially be bent to fit the crooked teeth and then gradually straightened to move them into alignment. In order to do that, the wires were tied in with smaller wires, which probably felt a lot as if they were being cranked. Today's materials are far more forgiving and gentle. You could literally tie our modern wires in knots and they would spring back straight. The pressure they apply is much gentler than that of the old steel wires, more like gradual, gentle persuasion than severe arm-twisting!

"BRACES ARE UGLY, AND EVERYONE WILL KNOW I'M WEARING THEM."

This was certainly true years ago but not today. Today's braces are much smaller than they used to be and ceramic, tooth-colored braces are available, as well as removable, clear aligners such as Invisalign. We even offer completely invisible braces that are attached to the back of your teeth. Nobody needs to know you're in the process of straightening your teeth. They will simply notice the positive results.

"BRACES HURT."

Braces are still uncomfortable at times, but thanks to our new materials and procedures, the forces applied to move the teeth are much lighter and gentler now, leading to less discomfort. That's not to say there isn't an adjustment period. I tell all my patients that, yes, there will be a moment during the first week they're wearing braces when they believe getting braces was the single worst idea they ever had. But that moment passes quickly.

In the beginning, your teeth are sore (much like a bruise or a sore muscle), which usually lasts about two to four days, depending on the individual. As the soreness starts to go away, you've still got to get used to having these unfamiliar structures in your mouth. You have to get used to the feel of them, the hygiene requirements, the challenges of eating with braces—all of it. But human beings are wonderfully adaptable, and the weird quickly becomes the new normal.

Some people deal with braces better than others. I had an adult male patient in his sixties. He will remain nameless to avoid embarrassment. His wife called me in a panic after he'd gotten his braces. Anyone near the phone could literally hear this guy moaning in the background as she told me he was in terrible pain and needed to be seen right away. Of course I told her to bring him right in.

When they arrived, I could see immediately that he was in real discomfort. He told me he wanted me to take the braces off, then and there. I managed to talk him off the ledge, pointing out that if I were to remove them while his teeth were already so painful, it would be excruciating. I asked him if he'd taken the ibuprofen pills I'd recommended, and he admitted he had not. "Why not?" I wanted to know. "I don't like to take anything," he said.

I assumed my best "doctor's orders" tone and told him, "Before you leave, you're taking four ibuprofen pills (the same as an 800 mg prescription dose), and I'll touch base with you tomorrow. If you're still uncomfortable, we'll set a time to get your braces off next week." I put the four pills in his hand. I gave him a cup of water, watched him take them, and sent him on his way. The next day, I called to ask him how he was doing. I left a message because nobody picked up. I was a little concerned when I didn't get a call back. But five weeks later, he and his wife showed up for his next appointment, and he said not a word about the earlier, panicked encounter. His wife said to me, "I told him to take Advil. He wouldn't do it." Of course, the pain had cleared up entirely with the ibuprofen.

Over-the-counter anti-inflammatories are the most effective treatment, and really all that the vast majority of patients will need for pain. I always give my patients a couple of Advil pills to take before they leave with their new braces. I tell them, "You may think you don't need them. Just consider it to be doctor's orders. Take them even if you think you don't need to. You don't get a gold star for enduring unnecessary pain."

"ORTHODONTISTS' OFFICES AREN'T OPEN AT TIMES OR LOCATIONS THAT ACCOMMODATE MY WORK SCHEDULE."

Depending on what kind of focus a particular practice has, you can find many doctors offering extended hours. We open at 7:30 a.m., which accommodates both adults going to work and kids going to school. In our adult practice, we're open during lunch so that people can pop in during their lunch hour and get back to work. And remember that after your braces are on, you'll have to see us every six to ten weeks, and those appointments are going to be brief.

"I'LL HAVE TO BITE INTO THAT DISGUSTING GOOP FOR AN IMPRESSION."

Not anymore. Thanks to advances in 3-D scanning, we can create a virtual model of your teeth—no more goop, which made many people gag or feel claustrophobic. Any sort of appliances you need can be accurately made using these virtual models—even Invisalign or lingual braces—and there's no need for unpleasant do-overs as there used to be when part of the old-fashioned impression didn't turn out properly. Now we can quickly rescan a portion of your mouth if we need to. The process involves placing a wand with a tiny camera into your mouth, and it takes about five to ten minutes at most. Almost everyone says the same thing once it's done: "Wow, that was easy!" Not all practitioners offer this. If it's important to you, ask in advance whether they do. When the original technology came out, I first had to try it myself. I decided I'd never have another impression done.

"I CAN'T AFFORD IT."

If that's what's stopping you from seeking treatment, you're probably overestimating the costs. Depending on the individual and the treatment required, in my practice the costs range from around $2,000 up to about $10,000, and there are many choices available to you within that range. A very complicated case will take longer, so the costs will be on the higher end of that scale, but even then, you'll be offered options. For example, lingual braces, which are completely invisible behind the teeth, are your most expensive option, with other less expensive options from there. But it's pretty cheap when you compare it to getting a single crown, which can cost $1,000 to $2,000. Beautiful straight teeth are among the few things that will last you a lifetime if you take care of them, and having that smile pays a lifetime's worth of dividends. It's an investment you'll never regret. Remember too that, most of the time, you won't be paying all of that cost up front and the cost can be spread out over time to accommodate your budget.

When you go for that initial visit and exam, your orthodontist should be able to tell you exactly what the process is going to cost. The vast majority of orthodontists will give you a flat fee with everything included, from retainers to the follow-up visits you'll make for a year or so after your braces are off. You'll be offered some choices among the various appliances, and you may be offered some add-ons, but there's no scenario that involves the orthodontist saying, "Oops. You're a year in and, by the way, I need another couple thousand dollars."

Remember too that this is an investment in your general health, especially if, as an older adult, your teeth aren't fitting together properly. As you age, that problem can lead to teeth wearing down, teeth breaking, and other problems you don't want to have. You certainly don't want to spend your retirement years in a dentist's office.

And I can tell you that in my years in practice, not one person has ever said, "I'm sorry I did this. I hate having beautiful teeth." What I do hear is: "I took care of my kids. They all got braces, they went to college, and now it's my turn to take care of myself," and, very often, "I wish I'd done this years ago!"

I had one patient who was a total charmer, a funny, warm, delightful guy—with some of the worst teeth you ever saw in your life. He had a gorgeous wife, certainly a testament to his winning personality, but you had to wonder how the heck he ever got her to marry him with a mouth like that! His case was so extreme that, barring jaw surgery, I had to tell him, "It won't be perfect, but it'll be a lot better." He was happy to go with "a lot better." And he got quick results. Within four to six months, he looked miles better. He told me, "This is awesome. If I had known I would look this great, I'd have been willing to pay three times as much." I laughed and joked, "Dang it! I wish I'd known that."

"AN ORTHODONTIST TOLD ME NOTHING COULD BE DONE FOR ME."

That may have been true at the time when you were told that, but materials and techniques in orthodontics have improved exponentially in the last few years and much more is possible today than ever before. It's also true that different practitioners have varying comfort levels in terms of what they are willing to attempt. Even if an orthodontist has told you she can't help you, that doesn't mean another orthodontist will be unwilling to take on your case. Some cases are more complex and require greater interventions, such as jaw surgery. You may not be willing or able to go that far, but there are often other options to explore—as in the case I described previously—that can offer tremendous improvement.

You might still believe orthodontic myths that need busting. If you're not happy with the way your teeth look, you owe it to yourself to get your questions answered—and those myths busted. Any good orthodontist will be happy to answer all the questions you've got. Just ask.

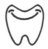

CHAPTER THREE

CAN THIS SMILE BE SAVED?

(And How Did My Teeth Get So Messed Up in the First Place?)

"Why are my teeth such a mess?" my new patient wanted to know. I had to explain, "This is one of those times when it's okay to blame your parents."

How your teeth and jaws are aligned is usually affected in large part by your genetic makeup. Even if your parents had perfect teeth, the combination of characteristics they passed on to you, when combined with environmental stresses, can leave you with teeth that are anything but perfect. If you've ever looked at pictures of the Hapsburgs, one of Europe's great royal dynasties, you're sure to have noticed the oversized lower jaw and underbite that characterizes many of them. Their genetic inheritance was complicated by the fact that they

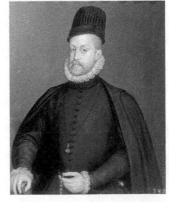

Philip II, Hapsburg King of Spain

commonly intermarried, but it's still a good example of a physical trait that runs through a family line. I've got a patient who had what she called the Gifford gap between her two front teeth, one she says she can trace through several generations via family photographs. On the other hand, I've treated three kids in one family, each of whom had completely different (and sometimes opposite!) problems. I worked on a pair of identical twins who had matching, mirror-image cross bites, which means the top teeth are within the bottom teeth. One of the twins had the cross bite on the right side, and the other had it on the left side. Clearly, genetics played a significant role in each of these cases, but it wasn't the only factor.

Environmental influences and habits are equally important. *Thumb sucking* is one of the most common. Let's say that one of those twins had been a thumb-sucker and the other had not; the thumb-sucker's teeth would be completely different from her sister's. A pacifier has the same kind of effect, although it's easier to get a child to give up a pacifier than it is to break the habit of thumb sucking.

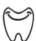

The vanishing pacifier: Here's a useful trick if you're trying to wean your child off a pacifier. Every few days, trim a tiny piece off the end of the pacifier. Within a couple of weeks, it'll be down to a nub, and your child won't be able to use it. Can't do that with a thumb!

Tongue posture habits can impact your teeth too. Tongue sucking is a habit some people develop when they're young: kids will put their tongue between their teeth and suck on it. Others will push their tongue forward and rest it against the teeth, putting mild but constant outward pressure on them. Those same people, as adults, will come to me asking, "Why do I have this space between my teeth?" Tongue thrusting has to do with how someone swallows. Ordinarily, when adults swallow, they position the tongue on the roof of their mouth behind their front teeth and bring their back teeth together. Infants have to protrude their tongues forward in order to nurse, and some adults don't lose that habit. So some adults have to keep their tongues protruded between their lips in order to swallow. These are tough habits to break because, most of the time, these people aren't aware they're doing these things, but once they become conscious of the habit and are given exercises to correct it, they've got a much better chance.

Occasionally, traumatic injury plays a role. It's possible for children or even an adults to break their lower jaw (usually the narrowest point of the condyle) without being aware of it—for instance, by falling and hitting the chin. Your chin is a strong piece of bone, but the force of such an impact is transmitted up all the way through the bones to the joint of the jaw, which is more fragile and may snap. Surprisingly, it's not painful and you might not notice any change in function. Ultimately, it will heal on its own, but it may not heal properly, or it may become shorter in the healing process. I've seen this in patients whose jaws are noticeably shorter on one side. If they remember having fallen on their chins, they usually dismiss the accident as no big deal. This sort of asymmetry can also be caused when the bone-building process goes awry—for instance, when one jaw grows faster than the other.

The third factor to consider is *time* combined with the challenges of genetics and environment. Whatever problems you might have had when you were younger will tend to worsen over time. I often see patients who tell me their teeth were beautiful when they were eighteen or twenty-one years of age. They'll show me pictures, and it's true. Their teeth may have been slightly crowded, but time worked against them to make the problem worse.

If teeth aren't properly aligned and nothing's holding them in place, they're going to move. If one tooth begins to cross over another tooth, they're just going to continue moving in that direction in a decades-long process. Similarly, if, as a child, you had a deep overbite, over time you'll start to see the bottom teeth getting crowded out because they have less room. Sometimes, when the bite gets deeper, the front teeth start spreading out. It's a combination of biomechanics and biology. When teeth are lined up, they're touching each other, and that creates a little bit of friction. If one tooth is slightly in front of the other one and the bone and the ligaments that are holding the teeth in place are constantly remodeling, the level of bone may change. Maybe you have periodontal disease, which has left you with less bone to hold your teeth in place, so they're more likely to move. Teeth are going to take the path of least resistance, depending on the pressures placed on them over time.

The other thing to be aware of is that teeth are made to erupt. It's just what they do. Let's say you have a bottom tooth that gets pushed backward so it's not in line with the others and it's not touching your top teeth anymore. Now that tooth doesn't have anything stopping it, so it's actually going to keep growing upward until it hits the roof of your mouth and stops.

HOW YOUR TEETH FIT (OR DON'T FIT) TOGETHER

There are problems that can affect your bite and that, in turn, will have an impact on how your teeth fit and function. I like to think of them as planes of space where you may have problems in the way your teeth fit together:

1. Front-to-back problems: protruding teeth, underbites

2. Top-to-bottom problems: the bite is too deep; the front teeth don't touch

3. Side-to-side problems: a cross bite

4. Perimeter problems: crowding, spacing

People are most often aware of the front-to-back class of problems because protruding front teeth and underbites are easily seen.

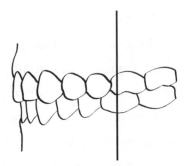

Class I Bite

Dr. Edward Angle, one of the pioneers of orthodontics, was the first to look at the way teeth were meant to fit together. He classified bites by the degree to which they matched the ideal or missed it. A Class I bite is the ideal. Everything's where it belongs: the top teeth fit nicely into the grooves of the bottom teeth, and the top and bottom teeth meet properly in the front. In a Class II bite, the top teeth are farther forward than the bottom teeth. Most commonly, this occurs because the lower jaw is not growing as much as the upper jaw. It can also be a result of how the teeth erupted or of habits such as thumb sucking, which applies pressure to push the top teeth out.

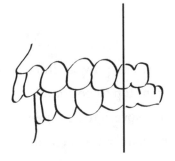

Class II Bite

Class III refers to a problem in which the lower jaw is more prominent

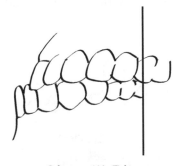

Class III Bite

than the upper jaw, and the lower teeth are in front of the upper teeth (the opposite of Class II). There's nearly always a genetic component to this. Sometimes the problem is created when the upper jaw is small and isn't growing forward as much as it would normally, but it also can be that the lower jaw is growing faster than the upper jaw. This is one of the more complicated jaw problems, and among the few things that respond better to treatment in young children than adults because the upper jaw stops growing when a child is about ten years of age, whereas the lower jaw continues to grow for as long as the rest of the body does, throughout the adolescent growth spurt. Depending on the individual, the lower jaw won't stop growing until the individual is between thirteen and eighteen years of age. If the upper jaw is problematically small, the window of time to correct that problem without surgery is between the ages of seven and nine, when we can put traction on the upper jaw, encouraging it to grow forward.

VERTICAL PROBLEMS

Jaws also grow at different angles, which can affect how your teeth fit from top to bottom. If you've got a square jaw, you're going to have a deep overbite because your jaws are almost parallel to each other and it's harder for them to fit properly. When jaws grow nearly straight down, you see an open bite in which the front teeth don't meet. A deep overbite is one of the worst things to leave uncorrected over a period of time because that's where I see adult patients who have literally worn their teeth down by two to four millimeters (or more!) over decades. At that point we're not just looking at having to correct the bite but

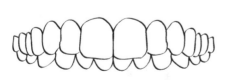

Overbite

also at significant dental work to restore the teeth. Parents may be tempted to shrug off a child's deep overbite since it "looks okay." And it may be fine for the next ten or so years, but in thirty to forty years, there will likely be problems.

There's a fair amount of confusion over the term *overbite*. I find that most people use it to mean that their top teeth stick out. Technically that's *overjet*. *Overbite* refers to how much the top and bottom teeth overlap.

The *open bite*, in which the teeth don't meet in front, presents a fairly severe problem both for your teeth and your long-term health because you can't bite through foods properly if your teeth don't come together.

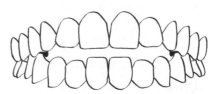

Open Bite

Tongue habits and thumb sucking can contribute to creating this problem, but often, genetics play the biggest role. In chewing, the front teeth are meant to guide the back teeth in functioning properly. An open bite means only your front teeth touch when you bite into something; your back teeth don't. They come very close, but they don't actually touch. When you shift that load entirely to the back teeth, you're asking them to do work they're not designed to do. They're made to grind food, and when they're forced to move from side to side, they're going to start to wear down and get flattened out, or even crack. That can lead to root canals and crowns down the line.

SIDE-TO-SIDE PROBLEMS

Ideally, the top teeth in the back of the mouth fit together with the outer cusps outside the bottom teeth and the inner cusps hitting the surface of the lower teeth. If you have a narrow upper jaw due to genetics or habits, the upper teeth may fit inside the lower teeth in what's called a cross bite. Again, this is a problem most easily treated in childhood, when the growth of the upper jaw can be guided and reshaped. Depending on the individual, it might be related more to how some of the teeth erupted, rather than to jaw growth, and it's better to wait until the

Cross Bite

child is twelve or thirteen years of age. In adults, if the upper jaw is narrower than the lower jaw, it can't be corrected without some kind of surgical intervention. The top teeth can also be completely outside the lower teeth. This is fairly rare and is usually due to a small and recessed lower jaw.

PERIMETER PROBLEMS (CROWDING OR SPACING)

Spacing or the crowding of teeth is often genetic in that the teeth are too big (or too small) for the space available in the jaw. Tongue habits or thumb sucking can also create spacing challenges. But with orthodontic treatment, we can line everything up. Perhaps 10 to 20 percent of patients will need teeth extracted in addition to braces because there's not enough room for their teeth in the jaws that they were given. If the mismatch in the jaws is really off and is creating a bite issue, fixing the jaw itself is the only option. There are limits to how much the jaw can be expanded side to side in any other way. People sometimes ask me, "Can't you make room by taking out wisdom teeth?" Unfortunately, teeth will only move backward with a lot of effort, and they don't move backward on the bottom at all.

Bad bites can have unexpected side effects, and sometimes I get to do a little detective work in ferreting out those effects. A few years back, I met Elizabeth, a lovely thirty-year-old with an open bite: her front teeth didn't meet. She had come to me because she wanted a prettier smile. In the initial exam, I noted that she had two molars on the bottom that had crowns on them, which surprised me. I said, "You have beautiful teeth, and you're really young. How did you get those crowns?"

She told me, "My dentist said I had a crack in my tooth, so I had to get a crown, and then the same thing happened on the other side." Almost as an aside, she mentioned that she also had some jaw pain, sometimes bad enough to give her a headache. Somehow, her dentist hadn't made the connection between her bite problems, the cracked teeth, and the headaches, but it was clear to me.

"That all makes sense considering the way your teeth fit together." I explained how the molars were being asked to do a job they weren't really designed to do, which was probably why they had cracked. "Sometimes, if your teeth are not fitting together, you're going to put extra pressure on them, or you may tend to clench your jaw to try and bring them together. That's where your broken teeth and those headaches are coming from." Once we'd done the work needed to correct her bite and achieve an ideal bite, she got lasting relief from those headaches *and* a prettier smile.

Now that we've gone over the many ways in which your teeth can wind up out of place, let's talk about what can be done to straighten them out.

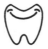

CHAPTER FOUR

BRACES, RETAINERS, AND ADDITIONAL APPLIANCES: HOW THEY WORK

I'd just gone through my proposed treatment plan with a new patient whose teeth were pointing in too many different directions. I'd walked her through the process, the timeline, and the outcome, the beautiful smile she'd always wanted but hadn't thought she'd ever have. She looked at me, her eyes like saucers. "How do you even *do* this?"

That's a question I hear a lot from new patients, and it always makes me feel a little like a Jedi tooth shifter. Patients' amazement at what we can accomplish is delightful to me, even when it's mixed with some skepticism that it really *will* be as easy as I tell them it will be. Some of them don't stop doubting it will succeed until their braces come off.

Typically, it's the adults who are the hardest to convince. "How can you move teeth? Aren't they solid? They *feel* like they're solid."

I explain, "You might imagine that the bone just grows right up into the tooth and holds it in place, but that's not actually how it works."

Your teeth are held in place by a whole network of tiny, infinitesimally short ligaments. Picture them as a net of rubber bands around the tooth that attach from the tooth to the bone. This network is called *periodontal ligaments.* (Learn that phrase and say it to your dentist. He'll fall off his chair.) We call it PDL for short.

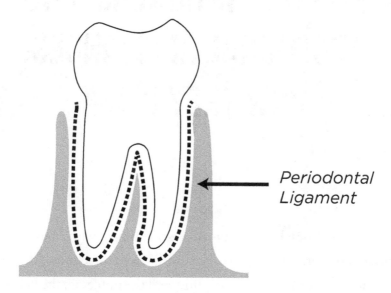

Periodontal
Ligament

The PDL is what makes it possible for a tooth to be moved. Because of this network, when you apply pressure on a tooth, the ligaments on one side are going to stretch, and the ligaments on the other side are going to get squashed. If you do that even momentarily, you can physically move a tooth and have it spring back into place. There's actual give in there.

Early in in my residency, the relationship between PDL and teeth amazed me. I remember a patient who had come in with a slight gap between her two front teeth. My instructor had me take a tiny little wire, tighten it up, and squeeze those two teeth together. Then we bonded the wire to keep the teeth in that position. I asked the patient, "Does that hurt?" She assured me that it didn't.

If you want to cause the tooth to move and change its position permanently, you apply force to the tooth, and you hold it there so that it can't spring back. Eventually, the bone on the side on which you're applying active compression sends out a message to tell the cells to make new bone and to take old bone away. The cells that make bone are *osteoblasts*. The ones that take the bone away are *osteoclasts*. I always picture those osteoclasts as little Pac-Men, going through and chewing up bone. The osteoblasts are following behind them to build it back up.

Of course, this process is not instantaneous, which is why it takes time to move teeth. Once the osteoblasts have rebuilt the bone, the stretch and the compression get equaled out again. It takes about four to seven days of steady pressure for this process to begin and for movement to start. And it can't be rushed, although patients ask me if we can't hurry the process up by applying more pressure. "Come on, Doc, crank it up! I want this done fast."

I have to tell them it just doesn't work that way. If this were rock rather than living tissue we were working with, that approach would work. In the case of teeth, however, if you push on them too hard what's actually going to happen is that instead of sending out all these useful little cellular messengers that serve as the wrecking crews and building crews, you'll squash everything and cut off the blood supply. Suddenly, all the bone and the cells on the compression side die. Then, because there are no cells there to do anything, you have to wait for the Pac-Men (osteoclasts) to come from the other side and, in effect, munch through a wall before the tooth can move. The fancy name for cutting off the blood supply is *undermining resorption*, and it actually slows down rather than speeds up the process.

There just aren't any shortcuts with biology. You can move teeth relatively quickly, but you can't move them faster than biology will allow. The body is smart. It knows what it's doing. We take advantage of the opportunity for movement that this network of ligaments creates and apply just enough force to gently push the tooth in the right direction, keeping that pressure steady over time. That allows us to maximize the biology to produce the movement we want as quickly as possible.

We've talked about how braces work biologically to move teeth. Now let's dig in to the technology.

"WHAT EXACTLY ARE BRACES?"

A set of braces is made up of two parts. One part consists of the *brackets*, which is the proper name for what's actually attached to your teeth. These are made of metal or tooth-colored ceramic materials. Some brackets have a built-in door that closes down to hold the wires in place. These doors make wire changes quicker and can make cleaning easier. Placing these brackets on each tooth is the most time-consuming part of getting braces, taking an average of

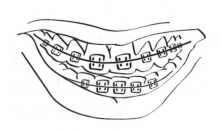

Brackets with Wires

fifteen to twenty minutes. Once they are attached, they remain in place for the entire time you're in treatment, unless you break them by eating something you're not supposed to.

The agent that causes the actual movement is the *wire*, which is placed into the slot in the bracket and goes from tooth to tooth. The wires are the active moving force and can be made of different materials that make them softer or stiffer. The wires and the ties that hold them in place are what we change and switch out as the process continues.

The wires moving the teeth can be attached to the bracket in several ways. In days gone by, the wire was held in place with a very small, very soft wire that your orthodontist would gradually tighten up. Those wires were replaced with small elastic bands, which come in lots of colors (generally more interesting to my younger patients, although I do have some adults who *love* their colored bands). Back when I had braces as a kid, I could have these bands in any color I wanted, as long as that color was silver! I remember my orthodontist father talking to a sales rep who was trying to sell him on the notion of colored elastics. "Why in the world would anyone want them colored?" my father asked. Clearly, he hadn't reckoned with middle school kids, for whom color choice is huge. They usually come in knowing what colors they want on their first visit.

The wires themselves can be made of different materials and come in different shapes and sizes. That variety lets me target exactly how much force I want to put on the teeth and what amount of control I want to have over a particular tooth.

The very first orthodontic wires were made of gold. If they were still in use today, they would be pricey. Gold is soft but almost too soft, and it's very easy to distort. Once it's distorted, it will move the tooth in a direction you don't want it to go, which is why orthodontists moved pretty quickly to using steel. Steel, even as very thin wire, is still relatively rigid. Fifty years ago, your orthodontist would have had to bend the steel wire to the crooked teeth and then manually straighten it out, which I suspect must have been what my patients were thinking of when they asked me if I were going to crank their braces. That manual straightening must have felt like cranking as the steel exerted powerful pressure on the tooth.

Over the years, inventors sought to improve the technology. Their ideas included taking a bunch of minuscule, stainless-steel wires and braiding them up. They were a little softer. Another idea was to take a little stainless-steel wire and put a bunch of loops in it. That made the wire longer, and the longer it was, the more flexible it was.

The last twenty or so years have seen giant strides in the manufacture of materials, and now we use wires made of nickel titanium. This is an amazing substance that I use whenever possible because it allows for light wires that give the continuous gentle force I described previously that creates the optimal biology. I can take one of these wires, literally wrap it around my finger, and then let the wire go, and it's going to spring back to the exact same shape it had before.

The particular alloy we use was originally developed by NASA as a material for antennas on rockets and satellites. You really can't have bits and pieces sticking out of a rocket when you send it up through the atmosphere, because those pieces will burn up in the extreme heat of the launch. But NASA needed to be able to put antennas on its satellites. So NASA researchers came up with this highly flexible material to manufacture an antenna that could be folded up inside a small compartment. Once the satellite got into space, the compartment door could be opened to deploy the antenna, which would pop back into its original shape.

The material itself has *shape memory*: it "remembers" the shape in which it was made, and it wants to return to that shape. That's what makes it so great for braces. When the wire is bent into the proper shape to fit in the mouth, it wants to be straight again. It's going to keep putting slow, gentle pressure on those teeth to line up as it straightens itself out. Such seemingly magical stuff was a kind of revolution for us in orthodontics because it meant treatment was now more comfortable and quicker than it had been in the past.

"BUT BRACES ARE SO UGLY!"

When you mention braces to most people, the metal mouth of yore is what comes to their mind. Again, however, technology has tremendously improved the look of them. Braces can be more or less aesthetic. It's your choice. You can wear the traditional *metal braces*. You can opt for the less obtrusive *clear braces*, or you can choose *lingual braces*, braces that are attached behind your teeth rather than on the front of your teeth and are thus utterly invisible.

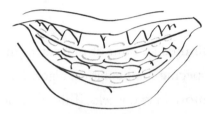

Clear Braces

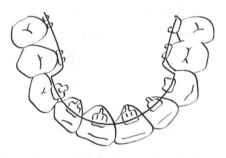

Lingual Braces

"ASIDE FROM BRACES, ARE THERE OTHER WAYS TO STRAIGHTEN TEETH?"

Aligners are an increasingly popular option for people who don't want braces. This process is completely different. To start with, aligners are made of special plastics and have different degrees of rigidity. As my magic wires do, they have some shape memory, but not as much. They have a little bit of elasticity to let them more gently move a tooth into place. Unlike wires, which can be adjusted, aligners cannot. That's why, typically, you'll go through a whole series of aligners during treatment. The number of aligners will vary from case to case, depending on how much movement is required, because each aligner has a limited amount of movement in it. Aligners are created using a very specific mathematical algorithm measuring how much a tooth can move in two weeks. This movement is calibrated during the planning and manufacturing phases, which are done digitally via computer. I'll talk more about the well-known Invisalign brand in a later chapter, but there are other makes of aligner as well. The idea of moving teeth with aligners has been around for a long time, and aligners have been created manually in labs for more than fifty years.

Aligners

Clear aligners are, essentially, a system of clear retainers that are preprogrammed with a specific amount of movement. Instead of wearing a bracket and wire system, which requires changing the wires to move your teeth, you wear a clear aligner that you can insert and remove easily. You wear an aligner all day for two weeks, except those times when you eat and brush your teeth. After two weeks, you'll progress to the next aligner, and then the next aligner, until you've reached your goal. It could take twenty or even as many as sixty aligners altogether to get you where you need to be.

Why might you choose aligners over braces? Two advantages are that you don't have any restrictions on what you can eat and you can brush and floss your teeth just as you've always done. Another advantage is that they're less obvious than braces. That said, if you're looking for maximum aesthetics—as in "I don't want anybody to know I'm getting my teeth straightened"—lingual braces that go behind the teeth are your best bet. Aligners are going to be slightly more visible.

The fact that you can put aligners in and take them out has a disadvantage, however: some people neglect to put them back in. As I always tell my patients, you're taking a bigger load of the responsibility on yourself with aligners. I'm doing most of the work on the front end to design the system to get your bite and your teeth back to where they're supposed to be. I've come up with a plan and provided you with the aligners. But I can't sit on your shoulder and tell you to wear them.

You have to be honest with yourself: will you be diligent and wear them as you're supposed to? I've had adult patients mull that question over for a moment and then tell me, honestly, "You're right. I'm not going to do that. Just glue something to my teeth. I don't want to be thinking about it. I want it out of my hands." That's completely valid. Other people will say, "That's perfect. That's exactly what I want." They're disciplined and they get it done. Self-knowledge is key. If you're among the latter camp, aligners are a great alternative. If you suspect you're not going to reliably follow through with wearing them if left to your own devices, then go with a different option and don't waste money on something you won't use. (Anyone out there own a treadmill they've "repurposed" as a laundry rack?)

There are a variety of extra appliances that sometimes come into play in the course of treatment. I talked a little in an earlier chapter about *expanders*. These are only used on the upper jaw, because its structure

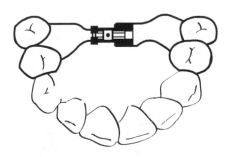

Expanders

allows us to push its two bones apart to expand it, and chiefly on kids because those two bones in the upper jaw aren't fully locked together until the kid reaches maturity. The lower jaw is impossible to change without surgery since it's just one piece of bone. Expanders literally get cranked because we're physically opening up space. We turn them a couple of times to expand them at the rate of about half a millimeter a day. It takes about two weeks for an expander to work to its full extent. We use them occasionally on adults, but they're not as effective as they are on children.

There are other kinds of expanders that are made of wires. One I use is a *quad helix*. This is an appliance for the upper teeth that is cemented in the mouth and has four active helix springs made

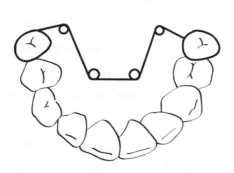

Quad Helix

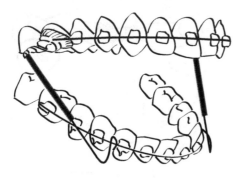

Bite Corrector

of steel wire. Let's say, for instance, that the teeth are leaning in and we want to push them outward from the inside, as in the case of a cross bite. We take a quad helix that's a little too big for the teeth, and squeeze it into place. Over time, it's going to expand out and move the teeth. This doesn't change the shape of the jaw itself but can provide enough correction to solve crowding problems.

Sometimes we use *bite correctors*. These are used to correct front-to-back-jaw alignment problems, primarily in Class II cases in which the bottom jaw and teeth are too far back from the top teeth. There are multiple kinds of bite correctors. The one I like to use is basically a spring that compresses. We hook it into place, and it stays in the mouth. This creates a light, continuous force—from the top teeth to the bottom teeth—that moves the bottom teeth forward and the top teeth back and thus corrects the bite.

An alternative way to correct the bite that almost everyone in treatment will use at some point is through elastics, which most people call rubber bands. When we move your teeth, each jaw moves independently rather than in concert. In other to make the teeth fit together properly, we've got to add something else. We might add one of those bite correctors that I described previously, but if it's a smaller movement we need, then a rubber band can be used, hooking from one jaw to the other so it can move the teeth in relation to each other to fit properly. The rubber bands can be hooked up in any number of ways to get the teeth to mesh together as well as possible.

None of these extra appliances that I've described are used throughout the entire course of treatment. They are things that come into play at a particular point—sometimes early on, maybe midway through treatment, or in the final months—and then are taken out again.

"I HAD HEADGEAR AS A KID. YOU'RE NOT GOING TO PUT ONE OF THOSE THINGS ON ME, ARE YOU?"

Consider this my solemn oath: no adult in my care is ever going to have to wear headgear. Period. Why not? Because it's just not necessary. Things such as bite correctors are going to accomplish the same goals in a much more discreet and less invasive and torturous way. Headgear *is* very effective for kids who are still growing, though. It works very well—but only on the top teeth. When used in concert with bite correctors on the bottom, we can accomplish a lot with a kid since we're taking advantage of that growth process.

"SO WHAT'S IT GOING TO BE LIKE HAVING BRACES? WILL IT HURT?"

I always tell my patients that when they come and get their braces put on, it's a piece of cake. Nothing is going to hurt. The worst part will be wearing those cheek stretchers—you've probably seen some— to hold the cheeks off the teeth as the braces are fitted because the teeth have to be thoroughly dry in order for the adhesive to stick. Back in the day, everyone had to have bands installed that wrapped around their teeth, and that was pretty awful for both the patient and the orthodontist, as the procedure was both difficult and time consuming. Now, thanks to a new generation of adhesives, we're able to glue smaller brackets to teeth. The adhesive can stick to tooth enamel or to porcelain if the patient has a crown. It can even stick to metal, depending on how it's prepared. The adhesive is formulated to withstand normal forces, but since it's going to be removed down the line, it can't be so durable that it won't come off when it's time to remove the braces.

Once the braces are on, or once the first aligner is in, it takes three or four hours for the teeth to begin to feel sore. I describe it as discomfort. It's not a sharp pain. It's more of an ache or a feeling of tenderness. This isn't a sign that anything's wrong. The process of moving teeth involves controlled inflammation, so the pain is a natural *initial* part of the process. When I finish installing braces on new patients, I always advise them to get themselves a nice meal because for the next three or four hours, they're going to be as comfortable as they're likely to be for the next few days.

For most people, the soreness lasts anywhere from two to four days, and the best way to deal with it is to take ibuprofen or naproxen, which are nonsteroidal anti-inflammatories (NSAID). Some patients will tell me they only use Tylenol. If, for some medical reason, a patient can't take an NSAID, Tylenol is fine, but it honestly won't work as well as ibuprofen. I tell my patients to take it consistently four times a day for the next two to three days, even if they don't think they need it. There's no point in suffering needlessly, and it's not as if the teeth will move any faster. Advil is going to make the transition a lot more comfortable.

Three or four days into this transition process, the teeth will stop hurting. That, however, is when the reality sets in. It suddenly hits the patient: "Holy cow, I've got this stuff glued all over my teeth. It's annoying. It's rubbing on the inside of my cheek. How in the world am I ever going to get these teeth clean? I get stuff caught in them. I go to lunch and I don't want to eat a salad because I'll get lettuce in my teeth."

This is an inescapable truth. There will come a day (usually about day six) when patients think they cannot possibly stand to wear these weird new things on their teeth another minute, much less for months. They will think that this is the single worst idea they've ever had in their life. What on earth were they thinking? They've got to get these things off. They're losing their mind. They think, *This is awful. I can't do this.*

There are very few people who don't hit this wall. For adults, I find that the frustration is most often about keeping their teeth clean, which seems so challenging at first. Everybody has that moment, and I'm not going to lie and say otherwise.

But the good news is that when patients get to that point, they're probably about twenty-four hours away from getting used to the new reality. They've hit bottom, and everything starts improving from there. Now they're going to begin to adapt. For most adults, after about a week, they're back on an even keel. For kids, it's usually no big deal. When I see my new patients eight weeks after they've had their braces put on, they all tell me, "It took a week."

The trick is getting past that first week and mastering the new techniques and tools needed to keep the teeth clean. The way you brushed your teeth without braces is not going to be the same way you brush your teeth *with* braces. One critical new area that demands special attention is the top of the bracket between the bracket and your gums because it's like a shelf on which food and plaque will gather. You'll need to use new tools as part of your hygiene routine. We have tiny little brushes shaped like miniature Christmas trees that let you get underneath the wires in between the brackets on your tooth. You can't really floss effectively because the wire is in the way.

The best option for keeping your teeth clean with braces, in my opinion, is to get a Waterpik water flosser. It does a lot of the work of ordinary flossing, getting in between the teeth and under the wires. My husband, who's a very meticulous guy, complained ceaselessly about the challenge of maintaining good oral hygiene when he first had his braces. I bought a Waterpik for him, and as soon as he began using it, he was fine. It was a portable version, and he took it everywhere with him. It's also useful when your braces come off, so it's a good long-term investment in your overall oral health.

"WHAT CAN'T I EAT?"

Adults with new braces are always concerned that they'll somehow break them or pull them off. And there *are* foods that are nonnegotiable no-nos. If you bite into a caramel apple, you're taking your life into your hands (in a manner of speaking). *Sticky foods* in general—

gum, taffy, gummy bears—will adhere to your braces, and by eating them, you risk either pulling off those brackets that we've glued to your teeth or pulling the wires of your braces out of place. I can tell you from experience that this will not happen on a Tuesday. It will happen on a Saturday, so you'll be stuck with that wire poking you in the cheek all weekend—a punishment that fits the crime.

Be cautious too with *hard foods* such as carrots. Instead of biting on your front teeth, you need to get into the habit of biting a little bit more toward the back. Cut your apples into slices.

Most foods are safe. You just need to be a little more mindful, and the majority of my patients quickly learn their limitations.

"I'M DONE WITH MY BRACES. DO I REALLY NEED TO WEAR A RETAINER?"

Short answer? Yes. Yes, you do. Why? The flip side of the orthodontic process is why retainers are critically important, although patients sometimes have difficulty understanding this. I can move people's teeth, but the mechanics that allow me to do so are *continuous*. Just because you no longer wear your braces doesn't mean the teeth are now set in cement and are never going to move again. The process that let me manipulate the biology so that I could move your teeth where we wanted them to go is the same process that allows teeth to shift back to where they were.

Why do they move back? Most of the time, the reason goes back to why your teeth were crooked in the first place. Teeth are somewhat stable. When we move them, we change the biological system. If there's perfect equilibrium, they may stay relatively straight. But more often, we've put the teeth into a position in which they don't really want to be. That's why wearing a retainer, whether it is removable or bonded, is essential to keeping those teeth in place.

I so often see adults who had braces when they were kids, whose teeth have subsequently become crooked again—sometimes a little, sometimes a lot. If you're in your thirties or older, your childhood orthodontist probably instructed you to wear your retainer for three or four years and told you that that you wouldn't need it anymore after that. I know my dad said that to me.

I have *no* earthly idea why anybody ever thought that was true. It makes no biological sense. Your retainer is a lifetime thing. If you wear it faithfully, your teeth will stay perfectly in place. If you don't wear it, they'll probably move. They might not—some people are lucky. But you're playing the odds, and the odds are against you.

There are various varieties of retainers. Some are removable while others are glued into place. These are often called "permanent" retainers, which is a misnomer (first of all, because nothing is permanent in life). They are glued into place with the same adhesive that we use to attach your brackets, and it can break.

Which type is better? There's a wide diversity of opinion on that, and if you were to ask ten orthodontists, you'd probably get ten different opinions. Some practitioners prefer a bonded retainer because, frankly, they want to eliminate the chance that the patient won't wear it. I hold to the opposite view. You've got to live with these teeth for the next twenty to fifty years (or more), so you need to take some ownership for maintaining them. A removable retainer puts you in charge—and you only have to wear it at night while you sleep, so many of the hygienic and other issues that a bonded retainer can create just aren't a problem. Also, if you have a bonded retainer, it could get broken five or ten years down the road. Chances are that by then you'll be nowhere near your original orthodontist. You go to a dentist who will likely tell you that you don't need it anymore. She takes it off. Now things start moving again.

Retainers themselves come in various iterations. The traditional ones that most people think of are made of acrylic and wires. I like them for kids in particular because they hold the teeth, but they're not on the tops of the teeth. Especially when a kid is still developing and the teeth are settling into place, some teeth aren't fully erupted, and the acrylic and wire retainer lets the teeth find their way into an ideal position. Also, this kind of retainer can be adjusted. It's like a "get out of jail free" card for kids' teeth.

For adults, I'll generally use a clear, rigid plastic retainer that's built to last and hold the teeth in place. Most adults have a tendency to clench and grind in their sleep. While their retainer isn't going to stop them from clenching and grinding, they're going to be grinding on plastic rather than enamel, so it serves as another layer of protection over their teeth.

Hygiene for a removable retainer is fairly simple: rinse it thoroughly when you remove it in the morning to avoid any build-up of the proteins from your saliva. You can brush it too, but rinsing off any saliva is the most important thing. A bonded retainer demands more attention. You'll need to use either a floss threader or a Waterpik in addition to brushing to keep it clean.

"HOW LONG WILL MY RETAINER LAST?"

Potentially, forever—but that depends on you. Serious tooth grinders can actually grind through them over a long (or short!) period of time. But unless you break it or lose it, you should be able to keep it for five to ten years at minimum and perhaps indefinitely. I actually had one of my father's patients come to me after thirty years to get his retainer adjusted. His teeth still looked great, by the way. I did a little tune-up on his retainer and sent him on his way.

I remember a patient who just goggled at me when I'd explained all of this to her. She said, "It's like you're one of those circus plate-spinners." And she wasn't far wrong. Orthodontists do have to take a lot of different things into consideration when they're planning a course of treatment. Fortunately, when I had my training, my professor—who literally wrote the book on orthodontics—taught us a very logical method for designing a treatment plan: the creation of a prioritized problem list. Everybody we see is going to have a set of problems. Some may have just one problem—for instance, crooked teeth. Some may have a whole batch of problems—for instance, cross bite and crooked teeth in combination. We have to prioritize those problems because correcting one problem may make another problem worse or more challenging to treat. In complicated cases we really *are* performing a balancing act, and in order to optimize our patient's results, we first need to determine which problem is the biggest priority for the patient. When I'm working with adults, we sit down and go over everything together so I can understand what their chief goals are and create the appropriate plan.

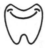

CHAPTER FIVE

THE NEWS IN ORTHODONTICS

When Allie walked into my office that first day, she definitely turned heads, and not just because she's a knockout, although I think that probably had something to do with it.

While she was checking in, one of our desk staff just had to ask her, "Aren't you on Channel Six News?"

Yes, she was—and as she explained to me a little later, her job as on-camera talent put her in an unusual predicament.

"I've been wanting to get my teeth fixed forever, but there's a clause in my contract that prevents me from changing my appearance, even a little bit. If I want to get my hair cut more than an inch, I have to get permission from the station manager first. And I *know* they're not going to permit braces—at least not visible ones."

My exam revealed that her case was a Class III, an underbite that put her bottom teeth in front of her top teeth, along with some asymmetry in her bite that meant the teeth just didn't fit together properly. If you looked closely, you could see it forced her chin slightly to one side, so this issue was as much about functionality as it was about appearance. Allie was a smart cookie and, good reporter that she was, she'd done her research before our meeting. She'd come to me because she'd read that one of my specialties was lingual braces, which are hidden behind the teeth.

"Nobody will see them," I was able to promise. "But I do have one concern. For at least a few days, your speech will be affected—maybe even for as long as a week or two."

That's when she told me that network stations like hers actually had speech therapists on call. She was able to utilize their services, and nobody could tell within a day or two that anything had changed in her diction.

Her case was challenging in that she required jaw surgery to fix the asymmetry, and the whole process took a year and a half. But the results left her even more beautiful, and it wasn't long afterward that she was out of that local news reporting slot and on to bigger and better things, working for one of the national network news programs in New York.

The fact is every aspect of the science of orthodontics has seen tremendous progress over the last twenty to thirty years, especially in terms of the materials used and the options they open up. No adult will ever be sentenced to metal braces, and there's honestly no reason to choose them. Ceramic braces work in exactly the same way, and the material is far more esthetic. And that's not the only thing that's changed for the better.

Back in the old days, the brackets that held braces had to wrap completely around the tooth because we lacked an adhesive that was both strong enough to hold them in place and easy enough to remove when the time came to do so. It wasn't until science came up with an adhesive that could adhere to the tooth surface that smaller brackets were possible—along with those nice, tooth-colored fillings that have replaced amalgam silver fillings.

That adhesive advance was the first in what came to be a kind of revolution, not only in aesthetics but also in the ease of installing braces. The brackets continued to shrink as orthodontists figured out the minimum area required to hold the braces in place and control tooth movement. Smaller brackets are not only less visible but also more comfortable, as they protrude less than the larger ones did. The early models of tooth-colored brackets, made of various plastics and composites, would discolor terribly, soaking up the color from whatever the wearer ate or drank. That's why we use impermeable ceramics now. Some are nearly clear and others are tooth-colored.

Lingual braces have the brackets that fit on the back rather than the front of the teeth. That means that unless you're howling with laughter, they're completely hidden. Not surprisingly, lingual braces were initially developed for people working in Hollywood in the 1980s. Those early lingual braces tanked because the brackets were so big they cut up the wearer's tongue, and fitting them to the uneven surfaces on the inside of the teeth was challenging. Because of this, the development of lingual braces was largely abandoned in the United States. Europeans, however, continued to work on perfecting them and were soon manufacturing smaller, custom-made devices.

Advances in technology and materials have made it possible for specialists to customize lingual braces to the individual wearer, which is both a great advantage and a challenge for the practitioner who doesn't do this procedure often enough to feel comfortable with the technology. If you're shopping for customized lingual braces, make sure that the orthodontist you choose is someone with plenty of experience in this area (and be very wary of any practitioners whose website features lingual braces as a treatment option but who then try to talk you into getting Invisalign instead, once you're in their offices). I often get patient referrals from orthodontists who don't have this skill set. Some will take a weekend course to earn a certification, but this is really an area in which practice makes perfect, so don't settle for less.

As with any braces, there are pros and cons to lingual. Most people will have a little tongue irritation at first and some degree of speech impairment for a few days to a couple of weeks until they adjust to having them in their mouths.

How invisible are they? One of my patients, Andrea, told me that when she'd run into people she hadn't seen for a while, they would invariably say, "Oh, you look great. You look different. Have you lost weight? Did you change your hair?" She never told any of them that she was straightening her teeth and none of them guessed. In fact, she even got married in her braces, and nobody knew.

Clear aligners are another alternative to traditional braces. They exert gentle, gradual force to guide teeth into place and work without brackets or wires. The technology was perfected by a scientist at Stanford who was wearing a retainer after his braces were off and realized that the same general idea could be applied to moving teeth. The first iterations were cast from a plaster mold of the teeth, but now the "mold" is a virtual model based on a digital scan. Based on algorithms predicting how much a tooth can be moved, the computer figures out how to get from A to B to achieve the desired outcome. The whole set of aligners is manufactured from that plan. How many aligners are used depends on how complex the case is. A simple adjustment, such as tweaking a few teeth that have turned in the front, might only require five aligners. A complex case could require sixty aligners.

One of the biggest advantages of clear aligners is that they are removable, which, as I said earlier, can also be a disadvantage if you neglect to wear them when you should. You can remove them to eat, so it makes hygiene a lot less demanding.

The best-known player in this arena is Invisalign, largely because this manufacturer had plenty of early venture-capital money to spend on promoting its product and perfecting its technology. Thanks to its early saturation of the market, Invisalign has become the Kleenex of clear aligners in that the brand name is synonymous in the minds of consumers with the product itself. But Invisalign is not the only option, and as its patents slowly expire, other companies are coming into that space. Now, with the advent of much less expensive and simpler 3-D printing and software, orthodontists are increasingly moving toward making aligners in-house.

One of my patients' favorite innovations is the *digital intraoral scanner* because it eliminates the need to take those yucky, gooey impressions that taste foul and make people gag. That technology was straight out of the Middle Ages. Yes, it worked well enough for the most part, but there were so many things that could go wrong with an old-fashioned impression. It was a fairly technique-sensitive thing, and some practitioners were better at it than others. Some were more likely to make patients gag than others. If it wasn't done right, it made an inaccurate mold. And if it didn't come out right the first time, there was no fixing it. You'd have to just start all over again and hope for the best, a depressingly primitive process.

The first digital scanners took about an hour and a half to make a scan, but the technology has raced ahead and now you can get a scan in two to ten minutes, depending on the level of precision required. Patients lie back as a wand is waved over their teeth—pretty painless and certainly a quantum leap beyond biting into a tray of goop. If any part of the scan isn't usable, it takes moments to go back and rescan a particular area. The level of accuracy and detail of these scans, once they're stitched together, is remarkable. We can do a lot with one of these models including using it in digital treatment planning, "virtually" moving teeth to optimize the treatment plan, and printing out customizing retainers or other appliances. We can experiment with different placements, installing virtual brackets and wires to see what will work best in treatment. It allows us a level of precision that just wasn't possible before.

Depending on the software we're using, we can incorporate x-rays and photographs of the teeth, or integrate a three-dimensional CT scan with real 3-D teeth so that we can see the whole picture. We're seeing more of these smaller CT x-ray machines in orthodontic and oral surgeons' offices. They're less precise than those found in hospitals, but they also deliver a far lower dose of radiation. I don't usually find them necessary in normal treatment planning in my own practice, but occasionally, when surgery is required, they're very helpful. If, for instance, a tooth hasn't come in properly and we're wondering exactly where it is, a regular x-ray would distort our view into 2-D and make it difficult to be precise. When we have a CT scan, we can see exactly, in three dimensions, where the tooth is. While this level of detail isn't required for most cases, it does help us to arrive at best-case treatment options for more complex cases.

Many companies are using virtual models to create precisely fitted braces, either with customized brackets and stock wires or with stock brackets but customized wires. There are hybrid versions too. Some lingual orthodontic systems now offer custom wires and custom brackets. All of these are designed to help create a greater level of precision. Orthodontists without these tools can, if they're good and detail oriented, get you to a similar outcome, depending on the complexity of your case. But they're not going to get there as directly. It's going to require more trial and error and tweaking along the way. It's a little bit like sailing. When sailors try to travel in a specific direction, they might have to tack to the right to catch the wind and then tack left—back and forth and back and forth. Eventually, they're going to get where they want to go, but not via a straight line. By contrast, digital treatment planning is like getting in a motorboat and going in a straight line. It's all proactive and pre-planned. Biology is not always so predictable, and there are inevitably times when things don't go exactly as we'd planned. But, more often than not, they do because we have the end in sight before we begin.

And progress continues. German engineers have actually built a robot that creates customized wires based on virtual models so that they fit a patient's teeth perfectly and accomplish what that patient needs to have done. Not only that, but the robots can bend wires that humans can't bend by shaping them under extreme heat during the manufacturing process. That lets us apply a light, continuous force with a customized fit that would have been nearly impossible to get before such technology existed.

Biology enhancers are an exciting—although somewhat con-troversial—new frontier in orthodontics. Some practitioners extoll their virtues and others dismiss them as modern-day snake oil. Speaking from my own experience, I've seen some promising results.

The least invasive of them is AcceleDent, a device shaped a little bit like a mouth guard that you put in your mouth and bite on. When you turn it on, it vibrates at a particular wavelength, and this vibration is transmitted into the bone through the teeth via the PDL. This vibration is intended to enhance the cellular response of the osteoclast and osteoblast, speeding up the process of moving teeth. It's used for twenty minutes a day. According to the manufacturer, this device can accelerate orthodontic treatment by up to 50 percent while decreasing the discomfort associated with treatment. That's difficult to quantify, of course, unless the patients use aligners, in which case we tell them to change their aligners every week instead of every two weeks. I use an AcceleDent device in my practice, and it does seem to enhance and accelerate the tooth movement, and there is no doubt that it reduces discomfort. Again, its effectiveness depends on how diligent the patient is about using it daily. Sometimes, people will get going with their treatment and become impatient for quicker results. I've found this device seems to speed up the process measurably, perhaps closer to 25 percent faster in my observation, rather than the manufacturer's claim of 50 percent faster. But such results are still nothing to dismiss lightly, especially when that can mean fewer months in treatment.

Another process, *accelerated osteogenesis*, radically speeds up treatment. While it can't accomplish as much as jaw surgery would, it can expand the jaw so that treatment can accomplish more than traditional braces can. This is a significantly more invasive method of treatment. A surgeon or a periodontist usually does the procedure. The first step involves going in under the gums and flapping them back. Then multiple holes are drilled into the bone of the jaw, and bone-grafting material is packed into those holes. This process creates a lot of inflammation that, together with all the bone-grafting material, makes the jaw substantially more responsive to any kind of orthodontic force. This not only allows us to move teeth faster but actually grows bone and makes the jaw itself bigger. As unpleasant as it sounds, it can take the place of more extensive jaw surgery. It doesn't require general anesthesia and can be done under sedation in an office.

One final innovation lets orthodontists get around the third law of thermodynamics, the law in physics that states that for every action there is an equal and opposite reaction. How? When we move teeth, pressure on one tooth is transmitted in an opposite way to the next tooth. But what if we had an anchor to pull against, one that can't move? That is where TADs come in. TAD stands for temporary anchorage device. This consists of tiny titanium implant screws—six, eight, or ten millimeters long—which we use as temporary anchors when we're moving teeth. Let's say a patient has crowded bottom teeth, but she's missing some molars behind them. It would be ideal to move those front teeth back, but teeth don't go backward on their own; they only go forward on their own. Adding this temporary anchor screw allows us to have something stable and stationary to pull against so we can move teeth backward into a space where there are no teeth, for instance. If there is something very specific we want to accomplish and we don't want to affect the other teeth, then these little temporary anchors can serve that purpose. They're not intended to integrate into and fuse to the bone as an implant does, so they're easily removed when the treatment is done.

The ongoing efforts by researchers and inventors mean that no matter what you've been told in the past about the limits of what can be accomplished with orthodontics, it's worth the time to get another, more up-to-date opinion now. What might have seemed like science fiction twenty years ago is fact today, and cases once dismissed as "hopeless" can often be successfully treated now.

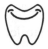

CHAPTER SIX

WHAT DOES IT MEAN IF I'M TOLD I NEED EXTRACTIONS OR JAW SURGERY?

"Wait! You are saying I need teeth taken out to straighten them?" Ben and I were going over his treatment plan together, and he did not look happy. "*Four* of them? Won't I have huge gaps?"

The hardest thing to explain to patients is why I'd even suggest extracting perfectly healthy teeth as part of their orthodontic treatment plan. Some people have enough common sense to look in their mouths and realize there's no way their teeth are all going to fit when they're pulled into place. Maybe other people in their family had teeth taken out when they had braces, so the idea isn't so jarring, but the patients who look at me as if I had just grown two heads are a little bit more challenging. And there are definitely some who look at me as if I'd just grown two heads. Ben was one of those patients.

I pulled up Ben's x-rays and explained to him that I was going to use the space the extractions created so there wouldn't actually be any gaps. He was really having trouble wrapping his head around that idea, so I gave him a big, wide smile.

"I had to have four teeth extracted when I got braces as a kid. Can you tell where I had teeth taken out? Can you see any gaps?" I smiled wide.

Ben peered at my teeth. "Uh, no."

"Neither can I—and I've never missed them. When we get to the end of your treatment, the only people who are going to know this ever happened will be you, me, and your dentist."

As I've said in earlier chapters, the structure of an individual's jaw dictates much of what we can or can't do in terms of moving teeth. That's why that structure sometimes needs to be altered, or teeth need to be removed.

"WHY WOULD I NEED TO HAVE TEETH OUT?"

Sometimes the amount of tooth structure you have does not match up with the amount of jaw structure you have—usually when your teeth are too large to fit into your jaw. Or you might have a mild jaw mismatch, and we want to camouflage your jaws and still make the teeth fit together. In the case of a child who's eleven or twelve years of age and still growing, we can usually take advantage of that growth to move things around without extractions. The jaw of an adult, however, isn't going to grow, so extracting teeth and creating space becomes necessary.

Maybe the lower jaw is a little recessed and the top teeth are sticking out. There's a slight jaw mismatch, but the face looks good, and everything's fitting together pretty well. One option would be to take out two teeth on top, usually the premolars (the teeth next in line past your canines, sometimes called bicuspids). By removing two teeth, I can pull back the teeth on top so that they meet properly with the bottom teeth. We don't change the way the teeth fit in the back, and we're not changing the way the jaws fit together. We've just camouflaged it, but because the top and bottom teeth now meet properly, nobody can tell what's going on.

If you have an underbite that isn't very severe, you might get two teeth extracted on the bottom, again the premolars, to accomplish the same thing. We're bringing the front teeth on the bottom back, so they now go behind the front teeth on top, and everything fits the way it should.

When teeth are removed to ease crowding, a premolar is generally taken from each quadrant because that makes everything match up. It's important to have teeth removed evenly because otherwise the bite will be off. The only time you'd have an odd number of teeth removed is when the bite is already off in some way. If the bite is off on one side, for instance, you might have one premolar removed. You might have just one front tooth on the bottom removed in the case where the lower incisors have become too crowded (usually we see this happen in older people).

Sometimes that's just the easiest way, and no one will ever know the difference, because the space is closed. If you have a slight underbite, the one incisor in the front could be taken out. If you're a symmetry freak, that will bother you, but nobody else is likely to see it. I actually had a patient who chose to have jaw surgery rather than have a tooth on the bottom removed because she couldn't handle the asymmetry. It was a good choice for her because it brought her upper jaw forward and really improved her appearance. When you move the jaw structure forward, you're stretching the skin over it more tightly, so it functions as a sort of facelift, a twofer!

"SURGERY? I DON'T WANT MY JAWS BROKEN!"

A bite issue is often caused by a big mismatch in the jaws—for instance, the lower jaw is so far back that only four teeth actually touch in the back. Alternatively, the problem could be an extreme underbite in which the bottom teeth are four or five millimeters ahead of the top teeth. Even a layperson may see it's not the norm but doesn't necessarily appreciate what is required to fix it. Within what we call the envelope of tooth movement, you can only move teeth a few millimeters forward or back, and that's usually sufficient for our purposes.

But if we're talking about a bite that's off by eight millimeters or ten millimeters, that's beyond the scope of what can be fixed by just moving teeth. At that point the only way to correct the bite is to address the underlying problem, which is the mismatch created by how the jaws have grown. Let me be clear here. We're talking about a very small percentage of cases, perhaps only two or three out of five hundred.

There are some cases in which we can camouflage the problem, and that's usually where extractions come into play. This is most useful for people who have a Class II condition—a recessed lower jaw with the top teeth protruding out—or sometimes a less severe Class III condition. The only problem with this approach is that you're starting to make some aesthetic compromises. Sometimes people choose to have jaw surgery because it's going to give them a better cosmetic outcome as well—for instance, if they've got a very recessed chin that they've always felt uncomfortable about. Surgery can bring that chin forward and dramatically change facial appearance so that the face looks a whole lot more balanced and normal.

In some cases, jaw surgery can also correct sleep apnea. A few months ago, I was visiting with a friend of mine whom I'd known since grad school in art history. We were sitting around, talking after dinner, when she suggested, "You know, you guys need to invent a better appliance for sleep apnea. I've got this appliance, and I've been wearing it, but I still wake up at night and I'm still not sleeping well."

I asked her, "Have you tried a CPAP machine?" She had, but it had not worked well for her, so she was stuck with this oral appliance that wasn't helping much either. As she talked, I looked at her as a diagnostician would. Even though we use x-rays and other tools, those of us who have been working in this area for years can look at people and get a pretty fair sense of their skeletal structure.

I said, "Laura, I do have an idea about what would probably cure this. I don't know if you want to go down this road, but I think the reason you have such severe sleep apnea is the relationship of your jaws to your airway. The most predictable way to cure that is with jaw surgery in which both jaws are moved forward. That would create more space between your spine and your jaws, so the airway opens up wider. That means that when your tongue falls back when you sleep, it won't close your airway."

She was amazed. Nobody had ever suggested that option, including an orthodontist she had consulted. For her, this surgery would have a profound health benefit because when the jaws haven't grown properly, it's not just bite or cosmetics that are affected; it can also be a huge life changer in terms of overall health.

Who do you see when your orthodontist recommends jaw surgery? You'll want to see an oral surgeon who has extensive experience in orthognathic surgery because there are a lot of oral surgeons who primarily take out teeth and only do jaw surgery a few times a year. They might do a fine job, but again, like anything else, you want the person treating you to be someone who does that kind of work all the time. This surgery would be a team effort between your surgeon and your orthodontist because it requires a combination of orthodontic treatment and jaw surgery. Some surgeons may want you to wear brackets at the time of surgery. They can be removed three or four weeks later if you have lingual braces or Invisalign.

The timing of surgery depends on a lot of factors. Generally, we first want to get the teeth lined up because when the bite is off and the jaws are off, we know the teeth will have moved to compensate for that. Once we put them in the proper position, they'll help to guide the jaws into the right place.

When people think of jaw surgery, their first worry usually is that their jaws will have to be wired shut. *They won't.* That used to be the case, but nowadays we have titanium plates and screws rather than wires, so everything's put back together nice and tight and you can open and close your mouth. Usually, you'll also wear some rubber bands because the muscles have to be retrained to a new position. You're not going to be eating hard food right away because, at first, you're not going to be opening your mouth wide. But your ability to open your mouth will rapidly increase, and strength will return. You can definitely eat soft things right away and work up to harder things, and you're not going to be sipping through a straw, unable to talk, with your mouth wired shut.

This kind of surgery is performed in a hospital under general anesthesia and comes with all the risks associated with any major surgery, so it's not a minor thing. Your surgeon will go over that with you. The worst part of the recovery is usually over after the first two weeks, and most people complain more about the swelling and the discomfort of chewing than about the pain.

One of my favorite patients is a guy named Mark. Mark is one of the happiest humans I've met, just a great, easygoing, nice guy. Mark also had the craziest mouth ever. When he came in to see us, he only had two teeth that touched, way in the back of his mouth. He had an underbite as well as an open bite, so the lower jaw was farther forward, and the teeth did not meet in the front. Astonishingly, he was not starving to death—humans are very adaptable. I don't know how he ate food, but somehow he made it happen.

When you have an underbite, it's not just that your lower jaw grew too much. It's usually that the upper jaw didn't grow far enough forward. Having both the upper jaw and the lower jaw too far back can contribute to sleep apnea, and Mark had some apnea issues. I had to tell him, "The only possible way to get more than two of your teeth to touch is for you to have jaw surgery. This is such a big mismatch that we've got to move the jaws into the right position." He wasn't thrilled about it, but he talked to the surgeon, found out exactly what was going to be involved with the jaw surgery, and finally agreed, "Okay, this is what I need to do for my health."

I usually see people about three to four weeks after their surgery's been done. That's still early on. They're past the worst, but they're not yet opening their mouths fully and are still in the process of regaining full function. But Mark came bouncing back to us in a week because he had to tell me, "I can finally breathe at night!" He was thrilled.

By the time he was out of braces, the transformation was amazing. He told me, "This has totally changed my life." He'd been taking all kinds of medications before—for his blood pressure and for high cholesterol, among other things—but now that his jaws were in the right position and he could breathe properly and sleep without interruption, he was off all of those meds. He felt better and was a lot more active in his life.

Sometimes patients come to me knowing they want jaw surgery. Alicia was one of them. Even though we could have accomplished a lot just by straightening her teeth, she wasn't happy with the way she looked with the rather mild underbite she had. She wanted her teeth to fit together and her jaws to be exactly where they should be. She had the surgery, and together, we produced a beautiful result. She was a really attractive woman anyhow, and now she looked better than she ever had. She was absolutely thrilled with her decision not to compromise.

People have their own reasons for doing things, and often it's not because I've told them, "This is the only way it can be done." Thanks to the Internet, people have very often done their own research ahead of meeting with me, and they know what they want changed. Some patients come in wanting to achieve the ideal, while others lean more toward the practical. I tend to favor the more practical approach. But it's important to me (and to you) that I always spell out all the options available because sometimes people will surprise me and say, "That's what I want." As long as I know they have all of the options and information they need to make an informed choice, I believe their wisdom and common sense will lead them to make the right decision for them, and I honor that choice.

Recently, I had an adult patient who, as a child, had her braces put on by my dad. Orthodontists working on kids do the very best they can to take advantage of growth to help the process, but sometimes it's not enough to make a perfect fix possible because there's just too great a jaw mismatch. My dad had achieved a good result with this girl, but as she got older, she still didn't develop the ideal bite. For some people it wouldn't have been a problem, but she had the recessed lower jaw and open bite that prevent the teeth from meeting in the front, and she had a lot of jaw pain, which was what brought her into my office.

"Your teeth definitely don't fit," I told her. "That could be part of it, but the pain could be coming from a lot of other things too. Maybe you're just clenching." We tried some conservative things, and my suggestion was a Botox injection in the jaw muscles to relax them. "Let's just do this as a diagnostic tool because, if it works, we'll know it was muscle pain. If it doesn't have any impact, then we'll know it's probably more to do with your jaw and could be because your teeth don't meet together properly." That turned out to be the case.

When she came back, I had to tell her, "Logan, we're looking at jaw surgery." She wasn't thrilled by that prospect, but as we were looking at her x-rays, I could see that she had a very small airway, and I asked her, "Do you have sleep apnea?"

She looked at me in surprise. "Well, I do snore a lot, and I feel really tired all the time. I've been meaning to go get a sleep study, but I haven't done it yet."

I nodded. "You probably do need to get a sleep study because that'll help in getting your surgery approved. But I'm sure your sleep problems stem from the way your jaws fit together."

That was enough to convince her to have the surgery, especially after both the results of the sleep study and a consultation with her surgeon confirmed what I'd told her. When she came back to see me afterward, the first thing she told me was, "I was breathing better from the very first day—and my jaw pain went away!" Now her teeth fit together properly, and her smile is even better.

Don't panic if you hear the words *extraction* or *jaw surgery*. Do ask questions because there's always a logical reason why these procedures are suggested, and your practitioner should be happy to explain it until it makes sense to you. Also, ask about other options, especially if you're not comfortable with what's being recommended. Sometimes the answer may be, "Nope. This is it," and other times, it may be, "Well, we have some compromises." Talk through the pros and cons.

Doing nothing is also an option if you can live with the problems you've got, but don't let unwarranted fears or an imprecise understanding of what's being proposed scare you away from needed treatment. You need that bond of trust with your practitioner, and if for some reason that isn't there, always, *always* seek out a second opinion.

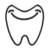

CHAPTER SEVEN

WHAT TO EXPECT WHEN YOU MEET YOUR ORTHODONTIST

"What's going to happen at my first appointment?" is one of those questions new adult patients invariably ask (with some trepidation) when they make that initial appointment at my office. Every practice has its own way of doing things, of course, but most of what happens in a first appointment at my office is similar to what happens at any office, so I'll describe our procedures when I talk about what you can expect when you meet your orthodontist.

Typically, we allocate an hour for an initial appointment. When you come into my new office for adults, I'll come out, introduce myself, and explain, "Here's what's going to happen. You're going to meet our new patient coordinator, who'll ask you a few questions about what you're looking to accomplish. We're going to take pictures and x-rays. All of that will take about twenty minutes. After that, you and I will sit down and discuss your treatment options and my recommendations."

At that talk-through, I'll give you a quick overview of your x-rays plus the overall health of your teeth. We use an x-ray called a lateral ceph that allows me to view the underlying structures to analyze how your jaws have grown and to look at where the teeth are placed within the bone. That helps me to figure out what's going on and why your teeth are where they are. We'll also go over your photos, and I'll explain to you what I'm seeing from a clinical point of view.

Some cases are fairly straightforward—"Oh, you don't like this gap here." But if yours is more complicated—for instance, if you have some significant bite issues—we'll discuss your goals because that's going to tell us where to focus your treatment plan, and I want you to know all your options. Usually, the more complicated the case is, the more options there are.

"WHAT IF I ALREADY KNOW WHAT I WANT TO GET DONE?"

Often people have a very clear-cut idea of what they want to accomplish. Sometimes those goals are complicated by other factors the patient can't see. One young woman who came to see me recently was a case in point: she had a gap between her two front teeth that she wanted to close. But there were other things going on too that made the case more complex than it appeared. Her lower jaw had grown a little further forward than the upper (Class III) and her top teeth were angled forward and protruding out. She just wanted that space closed, but putting braces on her would either have failed or would have left her functionally worse off than she already was. What looked to her as though it ought to be a fairly straightforward process was actually going to require extractions as well as pulling her teeth back into a position where I could get them to meet and overlap properly.

It was not what she was expecting or hoping to hear, I could tell. But there are some situations in which the physics and the geometry just aren't in our favor. That's when more complicated conversations are necessary, and people need time to process the information. When that's the case, I really work to help patients understand the issues so they can make their best-informed choice.

When the case is simpler, we move pretty quickly to discussing the available treatment options, whether they are clear brackets, Invisalign, lingual braces, or a mix of all of the above. I encourage patients to ask questions and help them to make a knowledgeable choice. Once we have a plan, I can tell them how long it's going to take, and at that point, I'll be able to tell them exactly what we're looking at, cost-wise. That conversation takes about forty-five minutes, but there's a whole lot of information to be reviewed, everything a patient needs to know to make a sound decision and move forward.

Most, if not all, people want two questions answered clearly: how long will it take, and how much will it cost? You should get answers to both of those questions at that first meeting. Your orthodontist should encourage you to ask questions and proactively offer information. If he or she tells you that what you want is impossible to accomplish, that may or may not be true. The fact is that some practitioners are more or less comfortable with various techniques, and even if your orthodontist tells you, "I can't do it that way," someone else might be able to. I hear this kind of story fairly frequently from patients who come to me for lingual braces after having been told no by other practitioners. The fact is if you sample five orthodontists, there will be some cases that all of them treat the same way. But there will be other cases in which you will get five different variations in treatment plans, and chances are they will each be valid. That's because it's not just science we're talking about. Artistry and a degree of personal judgment are involved too.

"SHOULD I GET A SECOND OPINION BEFORE I MAKE A DECISION?"

Some people feel duty bound to get multiple opinions, but my feeling is that if you like the first practitioner you meet, and you like his or her office, and you're being offered what sounds like a reasonable course of treatment, then getting multiple opinions is probably a waste of your time (and the doctors'). It ultimately comes down to trust; do you feel good about this person? Given that you're looking at a significant investment, you should feel quite good, and if anything about the office or the practitioner is making you uneasy, you should ask more questions or go someplace else. Also, ask questions about the technologies used—for instance, does the orthodontist take impressions, or does he or she scan? Scanning is not something every office is going to have available, because not every practice has made the investment in the equipment. A practice where everything is digitally planned is greatly beneficial to patients.

If you feel you're being rushed to make a decision, or the practitioner isn't listening to you, that's not ideal. There are times when I know that what people tell me they want can't be done. But I still hear them out, and I take the time to explain why a particular approach isn't as simple as it may initially appear. Some old-school doctors can come across as rather dictatorial: "Here's what we're going to do and how we're going to do it." That doesn't sit well with a lot people, though it is honestly more of a reflection of the doctors' chair-side manner than of their expertise.

I think you have a right to expect more. You should find somebody who's listening to your concerns because if they're not listening to you the first day you're in their office, and they're trying to gain you as a patient, you can be darn sure they won't suddenly start listening to you later.

"WHY MIGHT YOU RECOMMEND ONE PARTICULAR APPLIANCE OVER ANOTHER?"

My recommendations are influenced to some extent by what people tell me, which is why I think it's important to listen. For instance, if people want braces but add, "I'm worried about being able to keep my teeth clean," I might tell them, "If that's your biggest concern, then let's talk about the Invisalign device because you can remove it, so brushing and flossing stay the same."

Once your questions have been voiced and satisfactorily addressed, we nail down a treatment plan and discuss cost. The cost is going to be based primarily on the complexity and length of treatment as well as the kind of appliance you need and/or want. Ceramics are going to be more expensive than metals because the brackets themselves are more expensive to manufacture. Invisalign is more expensive still because it comes with the additional lab costs that we absorb. Usually, lingual braces are the most expensive option.

"WILL I HAVE TO PAY FOR EVERYTHING UP FRONT?"

At our practice, the answer is no, and we'll help you to come up with the best plan for your particular situation. Our new patient coordinator will go over your payment options. Fees can be paid over time, and she'll explain what your insurance will cover and what other options there are. Most practices offer a discount if you pay up front. Some may offer the option to extend payment past treatment time, with a small amount of interest added in. If the treatment is very extensive and expensive, you could consider using a financing company.

Orthodontic insurance, unfortunately, is not always available for adults. Many employers' programs offer it up to the age of nineteen or twenty-six, but not for adult treatment. If you are lucky enough to have orthodontic coverage, there is a set amount called a lifetime maximum that insurers will pay out. Depending on your specific plan, it could be from $1,000 to $3,500, but keep in mind that insurance will pay no more than 50 percent of your cost. The insurance company doesn't care what sort of treatment you have or what kind of braces. It's a fixed amount. Most often, the payment plans are set up so the insurance payments go to the orthodontist. As the patient, you get that portion of the fees taken off the top. Let's say you had a $6,000 treatment. You had a $2,000 orthodontic benefit, so now you're only responsible for the remaining $4,000. That $4,000 is what you're going to be paying over twenty-four months. If your benefit is paid directly to you, you're responsible for paying the orthodontist, but the orthodontist should file your claims for you.

Another option is using your flexible-spending account, which can be up to $2,500 pretax, depending on what your employer allows. It's important to remember we're most likely looking at treatment that will spread over two calendar years, so you're probably going to be able to put in $2,500, use it, and then contribute another $2,500 and use that. Another option is to use your health savings account to pay for orthodontic treatment. With flexible spending accounts (FSAs) and health spending accounts (HSAs), you are paying with pretax dollars. So, effectively, you're getting 20 percent or 25 percent more bang for your buck. Most offices will help you figure out what's best for you, and it's rare to come across any practice that won't file your insurance claims for you and collect them on your behalf. I feel that's part of taking care of my patients and providing good customer service.

"WILL I GET MY BRACES AT THAT FIRST APPOINTMENT?"

What happens next during your initial office visit depends on your choices and the orthodontist's schedule. In my experience, adults fall in one of two categories: some of them have made up their minds and come in ready to get started the first day. They've already thought it through, they've made their decision to go forward, and they're good to go. That's fine, assuming there aren't any dental issues that need to be dealt with first. I do sometimes see people who want to have their teeth straightened when it's clear they haven't seen a dentist in years. Sometimes their teeth are a bit of a wreck, and sometimes they're not, but in either case, they need to have a dentist overseeing their regular dental care while we're doing orthodontic treatment. My job is not to clean your teeth or to make sure you don't have cavities. My job is to straighten your teeth. I can easily refer patients to a dentist, and once they've got a clean bill of health, we're ready to go. I have lots of colleagues and friends who are dentists, as do most orthodontists. I like to do a little matchmaking and get my patients together with a dentist whose personality and style I think they'll be comfortable with.

If there's no dental work to be done, then the only other limiting factor is the amount of time in my schedule. Some days I'm totally slammed, but usually, if it's something quick, such as a scan for lingual braces or Invisalign, we can almost always work that in if you're willing to wait a few minutes. I have excellent assistants, so we'll do our best to make it happen. Patients who've decided on braces have asked me if they can get them installed during the first visit. Yes, if there's time in the schedule for it, we can put your braces on that same day. The only exception is if we are using an appliance that requires the old-school metal bands with a bracket attached, such as a quad helix or a bite corrector. In that case, we'd need to put in spacers first, which are little rubber bands that slide between your teeth and push the teeth apart, so the next time you come in, the metal band slips down into place easily.

"WHEN WILL I NEED TO COME IN AGAIN?"

After that, the scheduling depends on what kind of appliance we'll be using. If you're having Invisalign devices installed, it takes about three weeks to get the aligners back from the lab. It's the same for lingual braces. We'll be putting those on three weeks after your initial scan. If we put braces on, I'll remind you to take your ibuprofen because there's no prize for letting your teeth hurt, and I'll let you know that it takes at least a week to get used to braces. We'll talk to you about your new hygiene routine, supply you with some samples, and probably recommend a Waterpik. Then we'll send you on your merry way.

"MY DENTIST TOLD ME HE COULD STRAIGHTEN MY TEETH. IS THERE ANY REASON I SHOULD CHOOSE AN ORTHODONTIST INSTEAD?"

Sometimes I'm asked what an orthodontist offers in terms of training that a dentist does not. After all, there are dentists out there who work with Invisalign and braces. Why not just go to one of them?

There are several reasons to choose an orthodontist, the first of which is education. Every dentist—including every orthodontist—has four years of training in general dentistry to earn a dental degree. That four-year degree technically qualifies someone to do everything, essentially, in dentistry. Obviously it's no substitute for practical experience—developing knowledge and skills—but it provides a license to practice general dentistry. Within the dentistry profession, just as in medicine, there is a whole gamut of different specialties, orthodontics being one. An orthodontist nowadays usually has three years of additional training. Part of that consists of classroom work, and a big portion of the training also involves treating patients, which is why the training takes three years. It takes time to treat people, and orthodontist trainees have to have the time and opportunity to treat a number of people to completion. The issues of concern in orthodontics are things that aren't even touched on in dental school—ever.

I'm not saying that general dentists can't do some very simple orthodontic procedures fairly well. But why would you choose to be treated by someone without that unique, in-depth, specialized education? I understand a patient might view Invisalign as just another product, like a can of soup you can buy off the shelf. You can buy a can of soup at Wal-Mart or at the corner store or at a gourmet shop. It's still soup, even if it costs a little more at one place versus the other. The problem with that analogy is that Invisalign is not soup and it's not a product. *It's a process* and the amount of experience and education of the person directing that process makes a tremendous difference. I've seen and re-treated failures caused by dentists who tried to treat people with Invisalign. A lot of times, these failures, which weren't really challenging cases, were caused by dentists who didn't understand enough about the biology of tooth movement or the bigger picture of how teeth fit together. It's like everything else: whatever it is you want done, you want it done by someone who does that sort of thing all day long. You're not going to take your Mercedes to the Toyota dealership. You're not going to ask your family doctor to perform your open-heart surgery. Experience is the best teacher, and there's a reason for calling dentistry a practice. The more practice you get, the better you're going to be. Sometimes a patient will ask me, "Can you take out teeth?" and I reply, "No. You've got to go to your dentist for that. The last time I took out teeth was fifteen years ago in dental school. You don't want me to take out your tooth. Yes, I'm legally qualified to do that, but it would be a really bad idea for both of us."

Part of the confusion among consumers comes from products out there they call "six-month smiles" or "fast braces." There are ways to accelerate orthodontic treatment, and I've talked through some of them in previous chapters. But what often happens with these so-called six-month processes is that the practitioner simply does whatever can be accomplished in six months and calls the job done. There are cases in which that might be sufficient for what you want to accomplish. But more often than not, it won't be satisfactory, and you're still being charged a substantial amount of money. Getting a truly comprehensive treatment from a specialist could take a little longer and it will cost more, but there is no comparison when you look at the value of the result. If your dentist tells you she can straighten your teeth, don't jump at it. See an orthodontist first. Understand what you're getting into before you leap.

One great family came to me after having some less-than-optimal experiences with orthodontic treatments performed by their family dentist. Their younger daughter was the first of the family to come to me for braces, after her sister had had an unsatisfactory outcome from Invisalign installed by her dentist. Soon after, the mom came in for a consultation. She was concerned that her front teeth no longer touched. Everything had been fine until she wore a bite guard made by her dentist. This appliance was made so only her front teeth touched at night, allowing her back teeth to erupt enough over several years that her teeth no longer met in the front. I told her we could fix it with Invisalign. She was a little wary, given her daughter's experience, but we got her started, the treatment went very well, and she was thrilled with the outcome. They also had a son who'd had braces previously but whose teeth had shifted, so I put him into Invisalign too, and we got a great result. The mom was floored. "Wow, it's just completely different when an orthodontist does it." It wasn't, of course, the tool that had failed them; it was the practitioner and the process.

There's a reason that it's illegal to call yourself an orthodontist if you don't have that specialized training. Remember that just because people advertise that they can put braces on you doesn't mean they should.

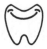

CHAPTER EIGHT

BUT AM I WORTH IT?

What makes people who know they need braces finally get off the fence and get them? For Kaleem, a terrifically engaging, high-energy guy, it was a wedding—*his* wedding—and starting up a new business. "I've got to get my smile in shape, Doc," he told me. "My folks offered to get me braces when I was a kid, but I didn't want to look like a dork. And I still don't!"

Kaleem had traveled 150 miles to come to my office because he wanted lingual braces, and now he was telling me he had to have a great smile—in six months.

I hated to break it to him. "You're not going to be done in time." He had much more work to do than we could possibly accomplish in that short a time, and one front tooth in particular needed to move forward pretty dramatically. His face fell, and I continued, "But I'll make you this deal. Wherever we are by the time your wedding day arrives, I can just put a bunch of bonding on top of that tooth. It will look great in your pictures, and then we'll take it back off after the wedding."

He smiled in relief. "All right, it's a deal!" So that's what we did. His wedding pictures came out beautifully, and he was thrilled. Finishing up the work took another year and a half, but he was committed. He'd realized, at this pivotal juncture in his young life, that his teeth just didn't match up with the bright future he had planned, and he was ready to fix that.

A big life change was also what steered Linea to my practice. A lovely woman in her sixties who'd been widowed a few years earlier, she was beginning to think about dating but lacked self-confidence in her appearance. Six months into her treatment, she met a terrific man. Six months after that, we were having a discussion about taking her braces off in time for the wedding! Fortunately, they were lingual, and she opted to keep them on.

Sometimes we don't believe we're worth it, but the people we love and who love us know that we are. Caroline, now in her sixties, had put up with a mouthful of crowded teeth for years before she finally came in for an initial exam with her husband in tow. We went over her options, and the two of them went home to talk it over. When she came back, she told me she'd decided on lingual braces.

"Okay, that's great," I said. "What made you choose lingual?"

She revealed to me that her husband had cancer. He'd been diagnosed several years previously and had been given two years to live, just over two years before. He was still doing remarkably well, but it was clear that he didn't have much more time. It was at his insistence she'd decided to get braces, and she chose the lingual kind because he'd told her he still wanted to be able to see her smile. Sadly, he passed away before she finished the treatment, so he never saw the beautiful final result, though his love and care for his wife lived on afterward every time she smiled.

Why do people wait so long to get the smile they've always wanted? The most common reasons are practical and financial. When people have kids, the kids get braces first, the kids have to go to college, the kids have to get married, the kids have to have whatever, and Mom and Dad come last, if ever. Sometimes parents will get braces for themselves when they bring their children in, but not often, unless they're relatively affluent. More commonly, Mom and Dad will come in when everyone else is done, the kids are out of college, and they can tell me, "I've done my job, I've taken care of everybody else, and now it's my turn."

The other thing I often hear is people expressing doubt that they're "worth it" or dismissing the idea of self-improvement as mere vanity after a certain age. They're concerned that they'll somehow look ridiculous for wanting to fix their smiles "at my age!" A woman once shrugged and said to me, "Well, I'm forty-eight now," as though she'd passed some arbitrary shelf-life, cut-off date and her looks, health, and positive self-regard somehow didn't matter anymore.

What I told her is what I tell a lot of people: "If your teeth are bothering you today when you're forty-eight, they're not going to stop bothering you when you're fifty or fifty-two or sixty-two or seventy-two." I know that's true because I see patients who are that age and who are still bothered by the appearance of their teeth. I think we sometimes have this idea that there's going to be a moment in the future when we'll give up all hope and not care anymore what we look like. I honestly don't think that ever happens, unless we decide to go and live as a hermit in a cave. We all want to look our best and feel good 'til the day we get in that box and go—and frankly, even then, most of us would want to have our hair done! Certainly, in my own case, the older I get, the more I am invested in how I look. There's a lot more maintenance involved than there used to be.

What people often don't weigh into the equation is how much better they'll feel about themselves when they're not embarrassed by their teeth. It's like the old story about the guy with a stone in his shoe. Rather than stopping to shake it out, he simply got in the habit of limping, a habit that eventually crippled him. Chances are that you're going to be limping along with bad teeth for a long time. If you're twenty-five, you could easily be looking at another seventy-five years with those teeth. Even if you're sixty-five, you're probably going to have twenty more years. That's a good long time to consider when you realize how much a great smile changes how you feel about yourself and how others see you every single day.

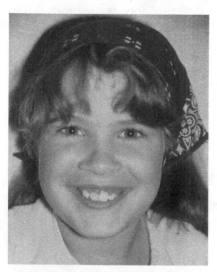

Before braces, age 7

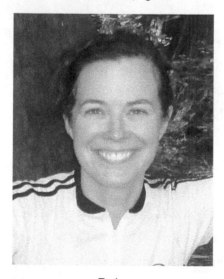

Today

When I was a kid, my teeth were absolutely awful, and I have the scary school pictures to prove it, complete with massive 1970s owl-eye glasses. For a kid with a mouth like mine, having an orthodontist for a dad was like winning the lottery. As soon as all my front teeth came in, he threw me in a chair and put some braces on me, starting out when I was about eight years old. I always joke that he was experimenting on me, but I understand it now. If my kids looked like I did at the age of eight, I'd be throwing them in the chair too. It's funny to admit it, but dentists are very conscious of how their kids look, and I get a lot of eight-year-olds whose moms and dads don't want patients judging their practices by their kid's scary-looking teeth. Ultimately, I had a full set of braces by the time I was twelve, so I have never had to feel bad about my teeth, not for a moment, or worry about whether people would judge me by my ugly teeth if I smiled. That was a tremendous blessing, as I came to realize in adulthood.

People always refer to me as a smiley person, and I have a really loud laugh. At the office, when I laugh, everybody can hear me. In fact, my laugh is so loud that it makes other people laugh. I have the confidence to know that if I'm approaching people to ask for something, I can give them a nice smile to smooth the way and make a connection. I just recently had a total stranger at a coffee shop tell me, "You have a beautiful smile." And that felt so good. It always feels good. It never stops feeling good. Knowing you have a great smile is like having a piece of self-confidence you carry around with you in your back pocket. Thinking about what I looked like at the age of eight, I have to wonder how much getting braces changed my path in life. My patients will often tell me, "I want my teeth to look like yours when I'm done." Given where I started out, that's quite a compliment to my father's work.

Whenever you do get them, how do braces change your life? It's back to the concept of the upward spiral I talked about in the first chapter. It's not just how amazing you feel the day you get your braces off and your teeth finally look great. It's that every day afterward adds to your new confidence. You see and feel the difference in how you interact with people, that day and every succeeding day. It's a benefit that continually builds on itself because now that you feel better about yourself, you're going to be more confident in every interaction. And in terms of long-lasting value, it's not remotely comparable to anything else you might do to improve your appearance. You may get your hair dyed, for instance, but it's going to grow out and you're going to have to get it done again. If you get a facelift, eventually it will sag and you'll have to get it tightened up again. But once you have your braces off, all you have to do is wear your retainers. A beautiful smile is like an antiaging device: it's never going to age as long as you preserve it. How many things in life can you say that about?

People put off getting braces because they shrug them off as "just cosmetic," as though having a positive self-image doesn't matter. Putting aside the derogatory assumption of a healthy level of personal pride implicit in this view, it is, in fact, important to have your teeth fit together properly so that you don't have functional issues. Imagine what happens to a machine whose gears don't mesh properly and you'll get the picture.

And to say, "It's just cosmetic" ignores the reality in which we live. You pick the clothes you wear and you pick the car you're going to drive. All such choices are, to some extent, about external appearances because they influence how we feel. How other people see us is central to our own reality, and perception effectively *is* reality. That's why when people contemplating braces for their child ask me, "Is this just cosmetic, or does she really need them?" I always say, "Well, nobody *needs* braces. You're not going to die of crooked teeth." Yes, you may suffer functional issues throughout your life because your teeth don't fit together properly, but for the most part, people get braces because they want to feel good about how they look—*and there's nothing wrong with that.* That's the best reason in the world.

In the first chapter of this book, I talked about how the smile is the most accurate expression of human happiness, joy, and pleasure, and a primary emotional communication with those around us. How can wanting to have a smile that makes you feel good and makes others feel good about you be written off as frivolous or mere vanity? When people hate their teeth, they cover up their smiles with a hand over their mouth, or they look away when they laugh, or sometimes they simply train themselves not to smile. I actually see patients who have to relearn how to smile after years of smothering their reactions. How can that be healthy?

It can't. It's not.

On the other end, I get patients who had braces as kids but then stopped wearing their retainers and are bothered by the subsequent shifting of their teeth. What's funny to me is that a lot of them tell me they spotted the problem thanks to the selfies they take for Facebook (thanks, Facebook!). Sometimes they're a little apologetic: "I know it's not that big a deal, but it bothers me." But my point of view is that if it bothers you, and we can fix it, why wouldn't you get it done?

My point is *you matter*. What you feel is valid, and it's healthy and good to address it. Make the appointment; have the conversation with your orthodontist. Let him tell you what's possible, and go from there.

New adult patients of mine fall into two camps: those who will make the decision to get started that day and those who will go home to think it over. Sometimes that second group doesn't come back for a long while. I've had patients pop up five years after that initial appointment to tell me they're ready to start. I think their hesitance is as much about psychology as it is financial. Sometimes there's an external motivation. For instance, divorce is a common reason for adults to get braces. People who've let their appearance slide suddenly see themselves as others will see them, and they want to look their best. Part of that is probably because when you're in an unhappy relationship, you don't look after yourself as well as you ought, but when you're out of it, your focus turns toward taking care of yourself.

I recall two patients who were typical of people who've finally made up their minds to get their smiles in shape. The first was a lovely woman in her fifties whose daughters had been patients of mine. She'd had braces as a child, but her teeth had shifted and, frankly, just didn't fit with her otherwise polished appearance. After waiting all those years and putting the kids first, she finally decided it was her turn. She's overjoyed with how she looks now, and she positively sparkles with confidence.

Patti was another great-looking woman. In fact, she was the star of a series of fitness videos. When she walked in, I recognized her but couldn't quite place her—until I realized she was the woman I'd worked out with all through dental school via those videos. I had to tell her, "Oh, my God! I used to see you every morning at 6:30 a.m." In addition to being in flawless shape, she had this great, smoky-sounding, sexy voice, and it was, frankly, hard not to hate her, especially at 6:30 a.m. in the morning. But meeting her now, I was delighted to discover what a sweet, funny person she was. Clearly this was a woman who was aware of her appearance. She came in to get Invisalign and was delighted at the results, telling me, "Wow, it was so much easier than I'd thought!"

Patti's reason for not coming sooner was that she was busy. As a teacher, she'd worried that it would be too challenging to fit the appointments into her schedule. Busy people imagine getting braces will be so much more disruptive to their lives than it actually is. Yes, there are definitely going to be some changes in how you take care of your teeth, and you do have to make those routine appointments, but it's generally much less of a commitment than you might think it will be.

I have a fabulous-in-every-sense older male patient whose picture should be in the dictionary next to the word *impeccable*. His suits are bespoke, his shoes are handmade, and his car cost more than most people's starter home. But somehow this supremely elegant man had gone through his whole life with really awful-looking teeth. His lovely wife had come to me and gotten her teeth fixed and was very pleased with the outcome. He'd met a few orthodontists in the past, he told me, and had been told he'd need jaw surgery, which was enough to put him off. But seeing his wife's transformation made him decide to give it one last shot. And that's when he came in to see us—at the age of eighty.

Fortunately, advances in the twenty or thirty years since his earlier initial consultation meant we could fix his smile without surgery. And he decided to go with it because he was starting a third career! If there was ever a walking example of why nobody should imagine that people could become too old to care how they look, he's the one. At eighty years of age he decided it's never too late. He ended up having a tooth removed and got his teeth straightened and fitting together, and finally, he got the smile he wanted. He finished treatment a couple of years ago but swung by the other day to get his retainer repaired—and to show me his beautiful new Porsche. Whenever people tell me they're too old, I tell them, "I have a patient who's eighty years old. How old are you again?"

How will having that great smile change who you are, beyond what you see in the mirror and what others see when they look at you? What I see in my patients is that they're just a little bit (or a lot) more confident; a little bit more assertive, a little bit more sure of themselves. There's a new spring in their step and a feeling of being ready to take on the world. I had one fellow who'd applied to medical school multiple times and been turned down. His career as a community college teacher had stalled. Frankly, he had goofy-looking teeth, and they had always been an embarrassment for him. After he finally got them fixed, his wife talked him into applying to med school one more time—and this time, he was accepted. That extra bit of confidence had been enough to propel him through the process, the "one last time" it took to get that happy ending.

Are you worth it? I think so.

IN CLOSING...

I've written this book because I passionately believe that everyone should benefit from orthodontics. Yet, too often, I hear adults say, "It's not possible," "It's too hard," "It's too late," or "It's too inconvenient"—every imaginable impediment. That's why, in addition to my two all-ages locations, I have a third office that's dedicated solely to adults. I started that office when I realized that nearly everything about orthodontic treatment is geared to what is convenient for a twelve-year-old and her parents. Our all-age office locations are near middle schools, and our hours are set to mesh with school hours. But what's convenient for a twelve-year-old and her mom isn't necessarily what's convenient for a working adult. The kid-centric location may not work, the times may not work, or maybe you just want to have a place that's more geared to you. My "grown-up" office is downtown, close to where my patients work. It's got work-friendly hours and a different feel that's solely focused on adult wants and needs. And my patients love it.

You can get a look at it on my website, www.drpitner.com. Design-wise, it's very clean lined and modern, a lot of white, with touches of wood and natural materials to make it feel almost spa-like. Unlike a typical orthodontist's office, which usually features a big, open room with a bunch of dental chairs, I've got frosted glass panels between chairs that give all my patients their privacy without making the office claustrophobic or dark. We're on the ninth floor and we overlook the grounds of the South Carolina State House, so there's a spectacular view to enjoy. If you're one of the many who have put off getting the smile they've always wanted, I hope you'll make an appointment and see my office—and us—in person. Whether it's because the kids came first, because someone told you she couldn't help you, or because you've hesitated due to the discomfort you assumed was an inevitable part of the process—whatever the reason you've avoided fixing what needs to be fixed—you'll find that things have changed for the better. It's faster, easier, and far more comfortable than it's ever been in the history of orthodontics to get the smile you've always wanted. Why would you possibly wait another day?

Printed in the USA
CPSIA information can be obtained
at www.ICGtesting.com
JSHW012056140824
68134JS00035B/3464